Clinical Studies Management

A Practical Guide to Success

Clinical Studies Management

A Practical Guide to Success

Simon Cook

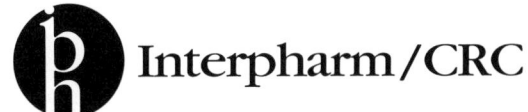

Boca Raton   London   New York   Washington, D.C.

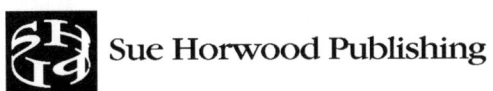

Library of Congress Cataloging-in-Publication Data

Cook, Simon.
   Clinical studies management : a practical guide to success / Simon Cook.
     p. ; cm.
   Includes bibliographical references and index.
   ISBN 0-8493-2084-4 (alk. paper)
     1. Drugs—Testing. 2. Clinical trials. I. Title.
   [DNLM: 1. Drug Evaluation. 2. Clinical Trials. 3. Practice Management—organization & administration. QV 771 C771c 2004]
   RM301.27.C66 2004
   615.5′8′0724—dc22
                                                       2003062073

This book contains information obtained from authentic and highly regarded sources. Reprinted material is quoted with permission, and sources are indicated. A wide variety of references are listed. Reasonable efforts have been made to publish reliable data and information, but the author and the publisher cannot assume responsibility for the validity of all materials or for the consequences of their use.

Neither this book nor any part may be reproduced or transmitted in any form or by any means, electronic or mechanical, including photocopying, microfilming, and recording, or by any information storage or retrieval system, without prior permission in writing from the publisher.

The consent of CRC Press LLC does not extend to copying for general distribution, for promotion, for creating new works, or for resale. Specific permission must be obtained in writing from CRC Press LLC for such copying.

Direct all inquiries to CRC Press LLC, 2000 N.W. Corporate Blvd., Boca Raton, Florida 33431.

Trademark Notice: Product or corporate names may be trademarks or registered trademarks, and are used only for identification and explanation, without intent to infringe.

Visit the CRC Press Web site at www.crcpress.com

© 2004 by CRC Press LLC
Interpharm is an imprint of CRC Press LLC

No claim to original U.S. Government works
International Standard Book Number 0-8493-2084-4
Library of Congress Card Number 2003062073
Printed in the United States of America 1 2 3 4 5 6 7 8 9 0
Printed on acid-free paper

"The cappuccino of project management guides: strong and to the point, but light and fluffy on the top"

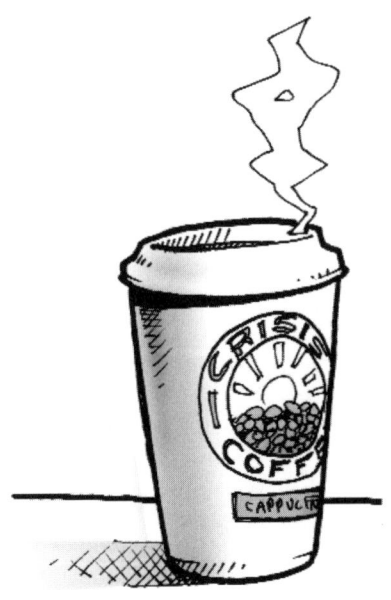

Author's Foreword

In the spring of 1989 I was busy with the life of an overworked Clinical Research Assistant (CRA), when the Director of Clinical Research walked into my office. She informed me that my project manager had just resigned, and that I was to take on his study responsibilities. My initial reaction was one of excitement at such a "battlefield promotion." Nevertheless, this was soon tempered with self-doubt over whether I had the necessary abilities to rise to the role.

There was no international Good Clinical Practice (GCP) at this point, and beyond quoting the 21 Code of Federal Regulations (CFR) 312 Guidelines to bemused Dutch investigators, I had no study management credentials. So flying by the seat-of-the-pants, I muddled through my first half-dozen studies, until someone had the foresight to send me on a management training course. In writing this book I am attempting to provide the desk reference I needed in 1989. This book was thus planned as an easy-to-read guide to the practical skills and methods required by project managers running clinical studies.

The book takes as its framework seven core themes: goals, budgets, time, resources, measurement, communication and training. There are also chapters on the drug Research and Development (R&D) process, Contract and Research Organizations (CROs), the clinical study team and Quality Assurance (QA) audits. Lastly, there is a true-life case history demonstrating how easily a project can go off the rails, and what can be done to recover the situation. It is thus a resume of how modern management theory can be brought to bear on the specialist demands of clinical studies.

I have not attempted to list all the various regulatory requirements in the countries of the world, but summarize the US and European Union (EU) scene. This book is for those wishing to sharpen their study management skills. They may already be project managers, or team leaders drawn from clinical monitoring, data management, study production support, laboratory, pharmacovigilance, statistics or medical writing. The book will be a regular resource for constant reference.

It is also hoped that CRAs, QA auditors, and CRO business developers will have an interest in dipping into this when delayed in airport lounges.

Having spent several extended periods working in the US, I know what it is like to be the token "Brit" on the team. There is much in the adage of "two nations divided by a common language." In the interests of maintaining the "special relationship" however, I have followed spellings used by Bill Gates rather than Her Royal Majesty. My European colleagues will also notice that I refer to "studies" instead of "trials", and Institutional Review Boards (IRBs) for Independent Ethics Committees, but rest assured there are plenty of Anglo-Saxon idioms along the way. Thus you should imagine me sitting on the windswept shores of Rockall as I pen this, halfway between Europe and the US.

So I hope you can find some pearls in the following pages to enrich your working day. For me, just sharing my "trials" has been immensely therapeutic. I thus dedicate this as a wreath to lay on the grave of that "unknown soldier" — the Project Manager.

To paraphrase Bob Newhart: "What would it be like if this complex and dangerous job was done by a bunch of 'non-experts'?"

Acknowledgments

The author wishes to acknowledge the following:

David Mitchell for his invaluable advice and input into the preclinical discussions in Chapter 1. David has worked in regulatory toxicity testing within the UK since 1978, for much of this time specializing in repeat dose toxicity and carcinogenicity testing and working primarily on pharmaceuticals. He passed the post-graduate Diploma of the Royal College of Pathologists in Toxicology (DipRCPath(TOX)) in 1989 and has held the Diploma of the American Board of Toxicology (DABT) since 1991.

Chris Brooks for lending the benefit of his experience in licensing medicines in the EU (Chapter 1). Chris has worked in regulatory affairs for 25 years, and is founder and partner of Quadramed, a consultancy providing a complete range of regulatory services to the industry.

Simon Parr for his distinctive graphic design and artwork, more often seen in British hobby and science fantasy magazines.

About the Author

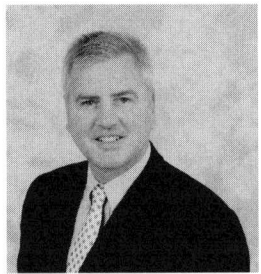

Simon Cook studied pharmacology at the University of Strathclyde, Scotland, and moved into the UK pharmaceuticals industry in 1984. Working initially as a formulation scientist, he quickly learned to "cut his cloth" between the needs of his marketing, production, medical and regulatory colleagues, "turning straw into gold, but without the straw."

As Good Clinical Practice became formalized in Europe, Simon returned to drug research, initially as a CRA, and then as an international project manager. During this period he spent extended periods living and working in both the USA and Belgium, gaining valuable experience in protocol development, GCP training, monitoring and management of Phase II–III studies, clinical study report writing, and the preparation of regulatory submissions. He was also responsible for CRO selection and management.

With his fingerprints on 50 clinical studies, Simon has research experience across all the major therapeutic areas, but cites his subjects of expertise as osteoporosis, dermatology, infectious disease and breast cancer. With over 15 years in the industry, he is now an independent consultant based in Berkshire, UK.

Keen on outdoor activities, the author is also a qualified canoe instructor and director of a children's charity camping organization. Drawing on these experiences during his working day, he believes strongly that the key to business success is in building highly motivated teams, and specializes in doing this on an international scale.

Abbreviations

ADME	Absorption, Distribution, Metabolism and Excretion
CANDA	Computer-Assisted New Drug Application
CBER	Center for Biologics Evaluation and Research
CDER	Center for Drug Evaluation and Research
CFR	Code of Federal Regulations
CHO	Chinese Hamster Ovary
CMS	Concerned Member State
CPMP	Committee for Proprietary Medicinal Products
CRA	Clinical Research Associate
CRF	Case Report/Record Form
CRO	Contract Research Organization
EEC	European Economic Community
EMEA	European Agency for the Evaluation of Medicinal Products
EU	European Union
FDA	Food and Drug Administration
FTE	Full Time Equivalent
GCP	Good Clinical Practice
GLP	Good Laboratory Practice
GMP	Good Manufacturing Practice
IB	Investigator's Brochure
ICH	International Conference on Harmonization of Technical Requirements for Registration of Pharmaceuticals for Human Use
IEC	Independent Ethics Committee
IND	Investigational New Drug
IRB	Institutional Review Board
ISO	International Organization for Standardization
ISF	Investigator Study File
ITT	Intention-To-Treat
IVRS	Interactive Voice Response System
KRI	Key Result Indicator
LOI	Letter of Intent to Proceed to Contract
MAA	Marketing Authorization Application
MRP	Mutual Recognition Procedure
NAS	New Active Substance

NDA	New Drug Application
PDP	Product Development Plan
PhRMA	Pharmaceutical Research and Manufacturers of America
PICF	Patient Information and Consent Form
PM	Project Manager
QA	Quality Assurance
QC	Quality Control
R&D	Research and Development
RFP	Request for Proposal
RMS	Reference Member State
ROI	Return On Investment
SAE	Serious Adverse Event
SAER	Serious Adverse Event Report
SAP	Statistical Analysis Plan
SOP	Standard Operating Procedure
TMF	Trial Master File
Tufts CSDD	Tufts Center for the Study of Drug Development
WHO	World Health Organization
WMA	World Medical Association

Contents

Author's Foreword vii
Acknowledgments ix
About the Author xi
Abbreviations xiii

1. Drug Development and Industry Trends 1
2. Contract Research Organizations (CROs) 19
3. The Role of the Clinical Study Project Manager 25
4. Goals and Standards 35
5. Budgets 47
6. Time 55
7. Resources 61
8. Measurement 67
9. Communications 71
10. Training 79
11. Surviving Quality Assurance Audits 87
12. Troubleshooting: A Case History 93
13. Conclusions 97

References 101
Index 103

Chapter 1

Drug Development and Industry Trends

FROM CONCEPT TO MARKET

This book is written as a practical guide for those managing or aspiring to manage clinical studies, but it is worth first putting this role in perspective relative to the entire drug development process.

The therapeutic uses of many of the drugs prescribed today were discovered by accident either from natural extracts (eg digoxin, aspirin, quinine, morphine, actinomycin D, vincristine, tubocurarine, penicillin) or as unintended side-effects (eg practolol, iproniazid, tamoxifen, minoxidil, sildenafil).

Since the 1980s, advances in cellular biology and genomics have allowed a more scientific approach. Greater understanding of the finer mechanisms involved in a disease process now allows the more strategic targeting of molecules which could act as potential therapeutic receptors.

A panel of *in vitro* screening tests (eg enzyme binding affinity, bacterial growth inhibition etc) is devised to select candidate compounds for potential drug activity. As data is collected, desirable atomic configurations may emerge, and computer modeling can then be used to further narrow the design towards the ideally shaped agent.

Nevertheless, the process is still extremely wasteful, and in excess of 5000 compounds will typically be screened in the search for one medicine.

The path by which drugs are developed today is dictated by the legal requirements of governments, most of which have licensing systems in place to control the sale and distribution of medicines. In broad terms, this is a sequence of cumulative information-gathering steps, each with a safety/benefit risk justified by the last.

Safety Studies

Once it has been concluded that a candidate molecule may be suitable for development as a potential new pharmaceutical entity, its progression towards successful registration will follow a closely integrated program of safety studies and human clinical studies. The "safety studies," mostly conducted using animals and always under controlled laboratory conditions, are primarily aimed at protecting those human volunteers and patients who will take part in

Test Purpose	Population Species (usual)	Sample Size[$]
Safety Pharmacology*		
Cardiovascular System[#]	Dog or Primate	4 - 8
Central Nervous System	Rat or Mouse	25 - 30
Respiratory System	Dog or Primate	4 - 8
ADME	Appropriate species	20 - 50
Single dose toxicity*	Rat and Mouse	40 to 80
Repeated dose toxicity (with toxicokinetics)		
14- or 28-day studies	Rat	80 to 180
	Dog, Primate or Pig	24 - 32
3-month studies	Rat	80 to 180
	Dog, Primate or Pig	24 - 32
6-month study	Rat	160 to 260
9- or 12-month study	Dog, Primate or Pig	32 to 48
Genotoxicity		
In vitro (Ames and CHO test)*	Bacteria or cultured cells	Variable
In vivo (micronucleus test)	Mouse	100 - 160
Carcinogenicity (with exposure data)	Rat and Mouse	600 to 1100
Reproduction Toxicity (with exposure data)		
Embryofoetal development	Rabbit	110 - 130
Fertility and embryonic development	Rat	200 - 250
Pre- and post-natal development	Rat	100 + offspring
Local tolerance	Rat or Rabbit	10 - 50
Metabolites tested in particular studies	Appropriate species	As above

[$]Sample size is a general indication only of the likely numbers of animals that may be utilized to provide the essential non-clinical safety data.
[#]May include assessment *in vivo* and *in vitro*.
*Required before first administration to man.

Figure 1.1. Safety Studies Conducted during "Conventional" Drug Development.

subsequent clinical studies from untoward and unpredicted effects of the new pharmaceutical or its metabolites. The type of animal studies conducted at each stage of clinical development will depend upon the amount of information already available from previous investigations, and the scope of the clinical study that will follow. Animal models of human disease may also be used early on in development to demonstrate efficacy prior to "proof of concept" in humans.

The non-clinical safety study recommendations for the marketing approval of a pharmaceutical usually include single and repeated dose toxicity studies, reproduction toxicity studies, genotoxicity studies, local tolerance studies and, for drugs that have special cause for concern or are intended for long duration of use, an assessment of carcinogenic potential. Other non-clinical studies include pharmacology studies for safety assessment (safety pharmacology) and pharmacokinetic Absorption, Distribution, Metabolism and Excretion (ADME) studies.

The goals of non-clinical safety evaluation include a characterization of toxic effects with respect to target organs and systems, dose dependence, relationship to exposure and potential reversibility. Initial safety information is important for the estimation of a safe starting dose for the early human studies and for the identification of parameters for clinical monitoring for potential adverse effects. Later studies are important, in conjunction with initial human data, for extension of the clinical studies program to longer duration studies and larger numbers of individuals.

A generalized list of the types of safety studies conducted at some stage during the development of a standard new chemical entity pharmaceutical intended for long-term use in patients of all age ranges is given in Figure 1.1. Short summaries describing each of the key non-clinical areas follow. Overall, the approach to animal safety studies and human clinical studies should be planned and designed in a way that is scientifically and ethically appropriate for the pharmaceutical under development. The standard approach generally applicable to situations usually encountered during the conventional development of pharmaceuticals may not be appropriate in all circumstances, and progression should be tailored according to what is known about the product under development and related products. This will invariably lead to "non-standard" approaches and the possibility of supplementary studies for many programs.

Safety pharmacology

Safety pharmacology studies investigate potential undesirable pharmacodynamics effects on physiological functions at exposure levels in the therapeutic range and above that may have relevance to human safety. Assessment of specific effects upon vital functions, such as the cardiovascular, central nervous and respiratory systems is considered most important. These evaluations may form part of standard toxicity studies but, because of their very specific endpoints and the need to look at dose levels in the therapeutic range, they are often conducted as separate investigations. For cardiovascular assessment in particular, because of a strong regulatory interest in QT interval prolongation, *ex vivo* and *in vitro* preparations are often used as supplementary or screening test systems (for example: the use of dog or sheep Purkinje fibers or ion channel systems). Supplementary studies may also be required to assess effects upon the renal/urinary, autonomic nervous, gastrointestinal and other organ systems.

Toxicokinetic and pharmacokinetic studies

Toxicokinetic and pharmacokinetic data should always be gathered along-side the main toxicology studies in order to put the significance of the findings in these studies into context for human safety and to validate the animal models. As development progresses, further information should be gathered on ADME in animals so that human and animal pathways can be compared.

Single dose toxicity

Single dose toxicity should be evaluated in mice and rats prior to the first human exposure by both the clinical and intravenous routes. These data are primarily to provide information and confidence on safety margins for that first human exposure and may also be useful in overdose situations.

Repeat dose toxicity

Repeat dose toxicity studies are conducted in advance of clinical studies for durations that are usually related to the length, therapeutic indication and scale of the proposed clinical study. In principle, the duration of the animal toxicity studies should be equal to, or exceed, the duration of the clinical studies up to a maximum recommended duration (usually six months for rodents and up to 12 months for non-rodents). These are expansive studies with collection and assessment of numerous toxicological parameters and extensive histopathology. The studies are conducted in two mammalian species, one of which must be a non-rodent. The selection of the non-rodent species is of paramount importance and should be based particularly upon closeness to humans in terms of ADME of the test pharmaceutical and its primary human metabolites. The species

Drug Development and Industry Trends

choice should be scientifically justified and may be made initially on the basis of comparative data for metabolism *in vitro* and subsequently supported by toxicokinetic and metabolism data *in vivo*. It may also take into account physiology and pharmacodynamics pertinent to the route of administration or the mode of action of the drug.

Local tolerance

Local tolerance should be studied in animals prior to human exposure using routes relevant to the proposed clinical administration. With the possible exception of products intended for dermal use, which may be administered by other than the clinical route in early toxicity studies in order to ensure adequate systemic exposure, this assessment is usually part of other toxicity studies. For pharmaceuticals intended for intravenous administration, however, it may also be important to study the effects of peri-venous and/or subcutaneous tolerance in case of problems with administration under clinical conditions.

Genotoxicity studies

Genotoxicity studies for the evaluation of mutations and chromosomal damage are generally needed and are conducted *in vitro* prior to the first human exposure. A test *in vivo* for chromosomal damage using rodent haematopoietic cells, with clear demonstration of target cell exposure, should be completed prior to the initiation of Phase II studies (although some Phase I facilities may, however, require to see this data prior to the first human exposure).

Carcinogenicity studies

Carcinogenicity studies are not usually needed in advance of clinical studies unless there is cause for concern; eg if suggested by genotoxicity data or what is known about related compounds. They are, however, usually required prior to marketing for any pharmaceutical that is expected to be given continuously for at least six months and for those used frequently in an intermittent manner for the treatment of chronic or recurrent conditions. For pharmaceuticals developed to treat certain serious diseases, carcinogenicity testing, if needed, may be conducted post-approval. The general requirements include one long-term rodent carcinogenicity study (usually in the rat) plus one other additional test *in vivo* for carcinogenicity (eg in transgenic or neonatal rodent models or a long-term carcinogenicity study in a second rodent species).

Reproduction toxicity studies

Reproduction toxicity studies should be conducted as appropriate for the population to be exposed. Outside Japan, men may be included in Phase I and II studies prior to the conduct of a male fertility study as long as an adequate evaluation of the male reproductive organs is performed in the repeated dose toxicity studies, but a male fertility study should be completed at the latest prior to initiation of Phase III studies (or prior to Phase I studies to be conducted in Japan). Women who are definitely not of child-bearing potential (ie permanently sterilized or postmenopausal) may be included in clinical studies without reproduction toxicity studies provided that the relevant repeated dose toxicity studies have been appropriately conducted. There are major regional differences in requirements for the timing of reproduction toxicity studies for women of child-bearing potential. In the US, they may be included in early carefully-monitored clinical studies without reproduction toxicity data being available, provided appropriate precautions are taken to minimize risk; including, for example, pregnancy testing and a highly effective (double) method of birth control. In Japan, assessment of fertility and embryo–foetal development must be completed prior to the inclusion of women of child-bearing potential using birth control into any type of clinical study. In the European Union (EU), assessment of embryo–foetal development should be completed prior to Phase I studies in such women and a female fertility study prior to Phase III studies. In all three regions, a study assessing pre- and post-natal development should be submitted for marketing approval, or earlier if there is cause for concern. In all regions, all female reproduction toxicity studies and the standard battery of genotoxicity tests must be completed prior to the inclusion in any clinical study of women of child-bearing potential not using a highly effective birth control method or whose pregnancy status is unknown. If pregnant women are to be included, all of the aforementioned will be required together with safety data from previous human exposure.

Juvenile animal studies

Juvenile animal studies should be considered when pediatric patients are to be included in clinical studies if it is considered that existing adult human and animal data (including appropriate repeat dose toxicity studies, all reproduction toxicity studies and the standard battery of genotoxicity tests) may be insufficient to support studies in such patients.

Phase I

Once the preclinical pharmacology and toxicology is complete, a picture will have developed in lower mammals of the dose required to achieve a therapeutic effect, its pharmacokinetics, and how this relates to the maximum non-toxic dose. While they can indicate trends, results from animal studies cannot be accurately relied upon to predict the human condition.

Thus first-into-man administration is a carefully controlled activity, generally performed in an intensively monitored hospital setting. This is known as clinical Phase I, and is conducted to confirm human safety/tolerability and pharmacokinetics at doses extrapolated from the animal data.

In order to reduce risk and maximize scientific control, the majority of Phase I studies are conducted in young, healthy volunteer adults. There may be exceptions to this however, particularly if the drug is expected to be toxic (eg cancer chemotherapy) or there is a known tolerance effect. Design and conduct will be in accordance with the Declaration of Helsinki, International Conference on Harmonization of Technical Requirements for Registration of Pharmaceuticals for Human Use (ICH) Good Clinical Practice (GCP) and any applicable national laws governing research on human beings. The experimental design will be placebo-controlled, often by treatment cross-over, but subject numbers will be small (10–20) and not suitable for statistical analysis.

Phase I studies are of two types. Stage 1 is a first-in-man single rising dose assessment. Volunteers are divided into cohorts assigned to receive progressively higher doses in a sequential fashion. The starting dose will typically be 10% of the minimum effective dose seen in animals (adjusted for human body weight). Regular blood and urine samples will be taken for 48 hours to build up a pharmacokinetic profile, and patients will be monitored and assessed for adverse events. The decision to escalate to a higher dose will be justified by acceptable results from the previous cohort.

Stage 2 studies involve multiple administrations. An optimum dose derived from Stage 1 will be given repeatedly at intervals of one drug half-life. These typically last for two weeks in order to establish steady-state kinetics, but may be longer if indicated by the drug class or an extended prescribing period. Once again, blood and urine samples will be taken at key time-points, and tolerability evaluated.

Phase II

Phase II clinical studies represent a progression from gathering information in healthy volunteers to those patients with the target disease. This is an important distinction for two reasons. First, the disease population may not be in the 18–30 age range typically assessed in Phase I. For example, diseases such as dementia, osteoporosis, postural hypotension etc predominantly affect the elderly, who also have impaired drug metabolism and excretion rates (ie atypical pharmacokinetics).

Second, patients who are experiencing the stress of a disease will have a very different drug adverse event (tolerability) profile from healthy volunteers.

Phase II studies collect safety and efficacy data in the normal clinical setting. This will be the first evaluation in man of the ability of the drug to treat the intended disease (proof-of-principle). Limited blood and urine samples will also be taken to confirm the expected pharmacokinetics.

A range of doses will be given to different groups of patients; bracketing the dose found in Phase I to achieve plasma levels which were therapeutic in animals.

Statistical comparisons will be made between the results of the different treatment groups. This then requires considerably larger population samples than used in Phase I, in order to overcome patient variability. Phase II studies thus generally involve 200–400 patients, contributed by many investigators working across different research centers.

Phase III

Phase III studies are large-scale multi-center experiments, usually conducted across many countries. Their purpose is to provide clinical safety and efficacy data which will be of sufficient quality to support approvals of a New Drug Application (NDA)/Marketing Authorization Application (MAA) by regulatory agencies (eg Food and Drug Administration (FDA), European Agency for the Evaluation of Medicinal Products (EMEA)).

Thus the disease definition (including severity), drug dose, formulation and administration regimen used in Phase III will be that which is approved for the marketed product. Optimum conditions should therefore be established before progressing beyond Phase II.

Characteristic of Phase III studies is experimental design which maximizes statistical power for population difference testing. The performance of the test drug will be compared against that of a standard therapy and/or a placebo. In order to eliminate sources of bias, treatments will be randomly assigned to patients, and the contents of the packs masked so that neither the patient nor investigator know which treatment is being taken (randomized double-blind design). To overcome variability, large population groups will also be used, typically 400–2000 patients, depending upon indication.

Product Licensing

Most governments regulate the distribution and sale of medicines by a licensing process embodied in their national laws. In the aftermath of thalidomide, the first country to comprehensively legislate for this was the USA in 1962, with the Food Drug and Cosmetic Act and subsequent amendments. The European Economic Community (consisting at the time of 6 member states) followed in 1965 with a Directive for member states to pass into local law, which described a national marketing authorization approval system for new medicines. In the UK, the Medicines Act was approved in 1968 and became operative in 1971.

USA

In the USA, medicine regulation is the responsibility of the FDA, or more specifically its Center for Drug Evaluation and Research (CDER) and Center for Biologics Evaluation and Research (CBER). In order to transport unlicensed drugs across state lines for the purpose of research in humans, the status of Investigational New Drug (IND) was created. Sponsors must apply for this with an IND submission. The regulations for this and any subsequent Phase I–III clinical research are set out in Title 21, Code of Federal Regulations Part 312.

The IND application should contain data on the animal pharmacology and toxicology, and any human results already gathered in other countries. Second, it will present chemical, manufacturing, stability and batch quality information. The submission will also describe the intended clinical development program, including proposed protocols, investigator details, and commitments to GCP principles. The FDA has a 30-day period in which to review the IND application for safety, and ensure that research subjects will not be exposed to unreasonable risk.

The clinical development must then be conducted under the terms of the IND approval, and may be stopped by the CDER if adverse event reports indicate a safety hazard. If all is well, the completed study data is then submitted as an NDA together with non-clinical safety and pharmacology results, chemistry and manufacturing information. A particular feature of the US system is that the sponsors are allowed to consult with CDER representatives prior to filing an IND. When NDA review is complete, the sponsor is given an opportunity to answer any questions, before a final decision is made. In 2001 CMR International reported that the median NDA approval time was 13 months.

European Union

In Europe, Directive 65/65/EEC requires that each member state legally authorizes medicines before they are placed on the national market, and sets out the standardized framework within which this should occur. This Directive outlines the pharmaceutical, scientific, quality, safety and efficacy criteria which should be met in order to grant a marketing authorization, and the format for the relevant application.

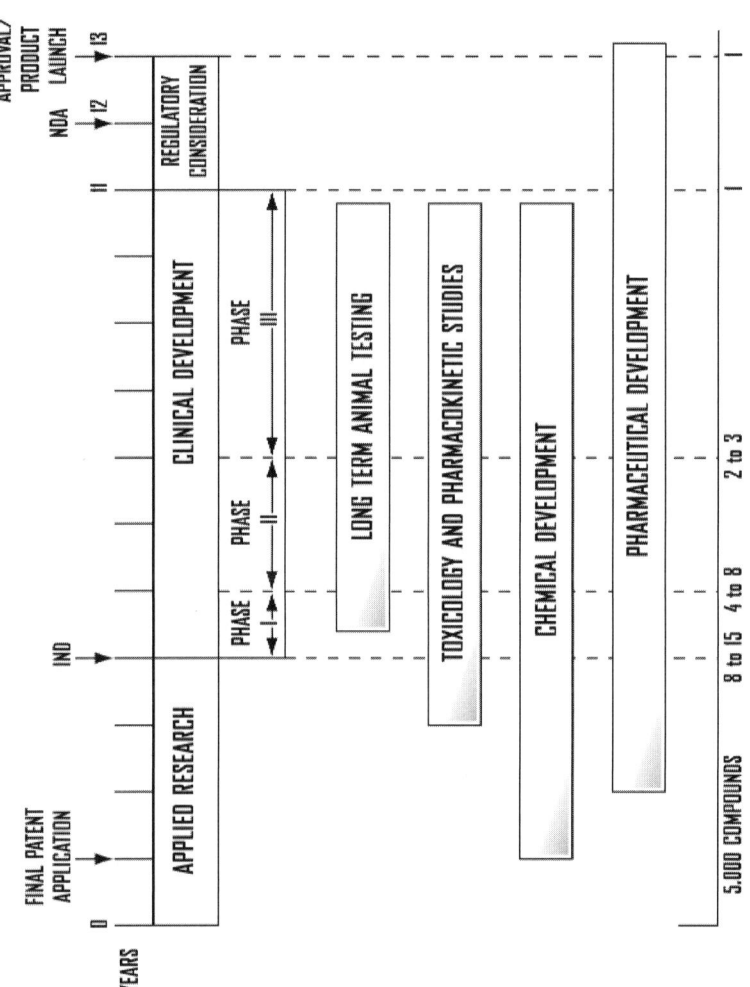

Figure 1.2. The Drug R&D Process.

However Directive 65/65/EEC did not set up a unified IND-type system for the regulatory approval of clinical study administration for unlicensed drugs. This has been determined individually by each nation, and ranges from a 60-day health authority review (Spain, Finland), confirmation of Institutional Review Board (IRB) approval (Belgium, Germany) to simple notification by import licence (Netherlands). A more recent European Clinical Trials Directive, 2001/20/EC, seeks to establish a standardized clinical trial application procedure to be implemented by May 2004. Although a number of implementary texts have been issued, at the time of going to press it is not clear how and to what extent member states will enact this.

The EEC has adopted directives since 1965 which have amended and extended Directive 65/65/EEC. These directives have developed the framework for regulating medicinal products, the data requirements and the procedures which may be used for reaching a decision on marketing authorization, refusal, revocation or suspension. Directive 75/319/EEC expanded the framework for medicines' regulation, particularly with regard to manufacturing and also established the Committee for Proprietary Medicinal Products (CPMP), a scientific review committee for multi-state and concertation procedures. These directives apply in all 15 member states of the EEC and have harmonized many aspects of the manufacture, sale, supply and registration of medicinal products for human use across the Community. The most significant development affecting the registration and marketing authorization of medicinal products since 1965 was the decision by the EEC Council of Ministers in October 1993 to establish the EMEA in the United Kingdom in London on 1 January 1995 and to introduce both decentralized and centralized procedures for dealing with marketing authorizations in the member states of the EEC. The EEC Commission has published a series of publications entitled *The Rules Governing Medicinal Products in the European Community* which are essential texts for anyone interested in manufacturing, selling, supplying and registering pharmaceutical products in the EEC. The centralized procedure is mandatory for List A products (recombinant DNA technology, gene therapeutics, monoclonal antibodies) and optional for those in List B (new chemical entities, products from human blood or plasma and innovative products). The sponsor must notify the agency 4–6 months in advance of its intention to submit. The review period for the initial CPMP opinion is limited, however, to 210 days, but there are clock stops within this while assessors are waiting for questions to be answered by the sponsor. In the case of an unfavorable opinion, the applicant has 60 days to present the grounds of appeal and the CPMP has a further 60 days to reconsider. Within 60 days of the CPMP opinion, the Commission prepares a draft decision which is made final after circulation to the member states and in consultation with the Standing Committee on Medicinal Products for Human Use. Once the final decision is made, the authorization is valid across the whole community. In 2001 CMR International reported that the median EMEA approval time was 16 months.

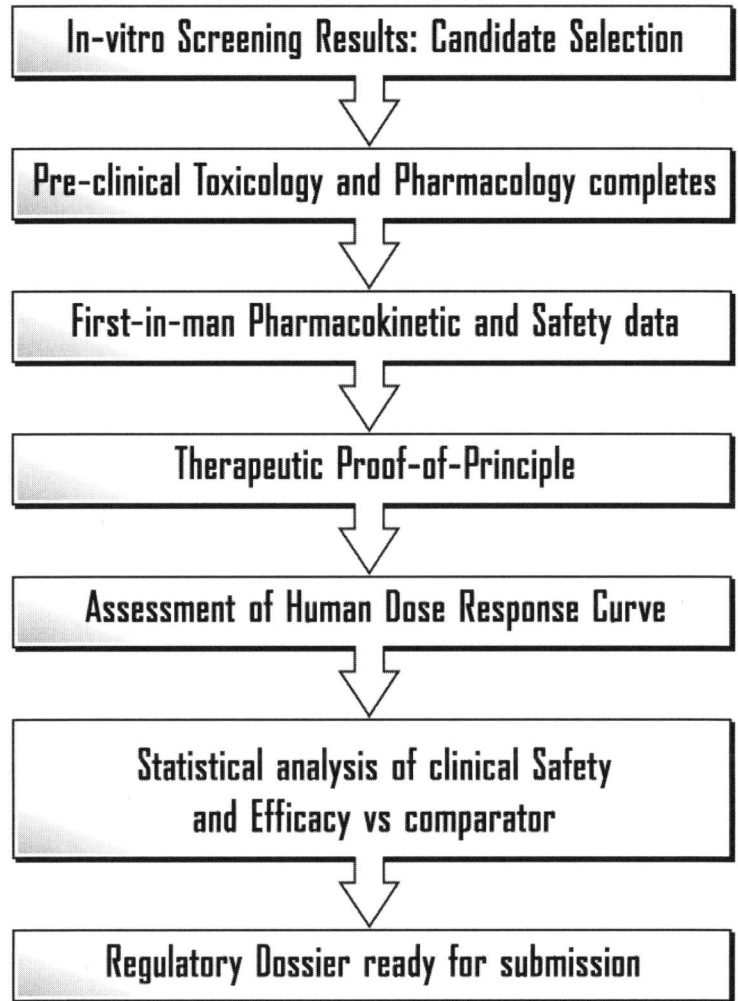

Figure 1.3. Strategic Review Milestones.

Since 1995, Directive 2309/93 has provided a decentralized route to obtaining EU marketing approval. Known as the Mutual Recognition Procedure (MRP), an applicant may first obtain approval in one country, call the Reference Member State (RMS), and then have the approval recognized by other regulatory authorities.

National approval of an MAA will take 210 days, plus clock-stops for responses to questions. To progress into MRP, an updated dossier is then submitted by the sponsor to the RMS authority. The RMS will then produce within 90 days an updated authority assessment report to be distributed to the desired Concerned Member States (CMSs). In parallel, the sponsor supplies translations of the product literature and submits the updated dossier to the CMSs. After a further 90-day period for mutual recognition, the CMSs then have 30 days in which to issue local product authorizations.

At 420 days, MRP is more lengthy and complex than the centralized route. However, it offers the advantage that marketing can begin in the RMS immediately on receipt of initial national approval. Nevertheless, it is less predictable for pan-European licensing, since delays can occur if a CMS raises significant questions or objections to recognition. The other side of the coin is that centralized approval is an all-or-nothing gamble with the EMEA. Proposals for modifying both systems are under discussion at the time of going to press. The original directive and subsequent Council directives were consolidated in 2001 into a single text in Directive 2001/83/EC on the Community code relating to medicinal products for human use.

Strategic Decisions

Putting it all together, the Research and Development (R&D) life of a drug follows a preset scheme determined by the regulatory authorities (see Figure 1.2). Lab discovery and animal toxicity/pharmacology tests are followed by clinical escalation through Phases I–III. Simultaneously, long-term non-clinical safety studies and pharmaceutical/formulation activities will be ongoing. The resulting data is then compiled into an NDA/MAA, and submitted to regulatory agencies for review. Figure 1.3 indicates the milestones for a strategic review of data.

At each stage along this path, financial commitment to the drug increases. Thousands of candidate molecules will be discarded in the search for success. This is not so much of an issue during the early screening stages, but the corporate risk associated with New Active Substance (NAS) failure grows dramatically as development progresses into the clinic (see Chapter 5).

In order to manage this accumulation of exposure, the product development team will run several parallel NASs. As the project progresses, the most promising will be advanced, as the weaker either fail or are "weeded out." This is achieved through a series of stop/go decisions at strategic points in the Product Development Plan (PDP).

At each assessment, the product development team will have to justify continued investment in the development of a potential medicine. This decision will be based on the following six criteria:

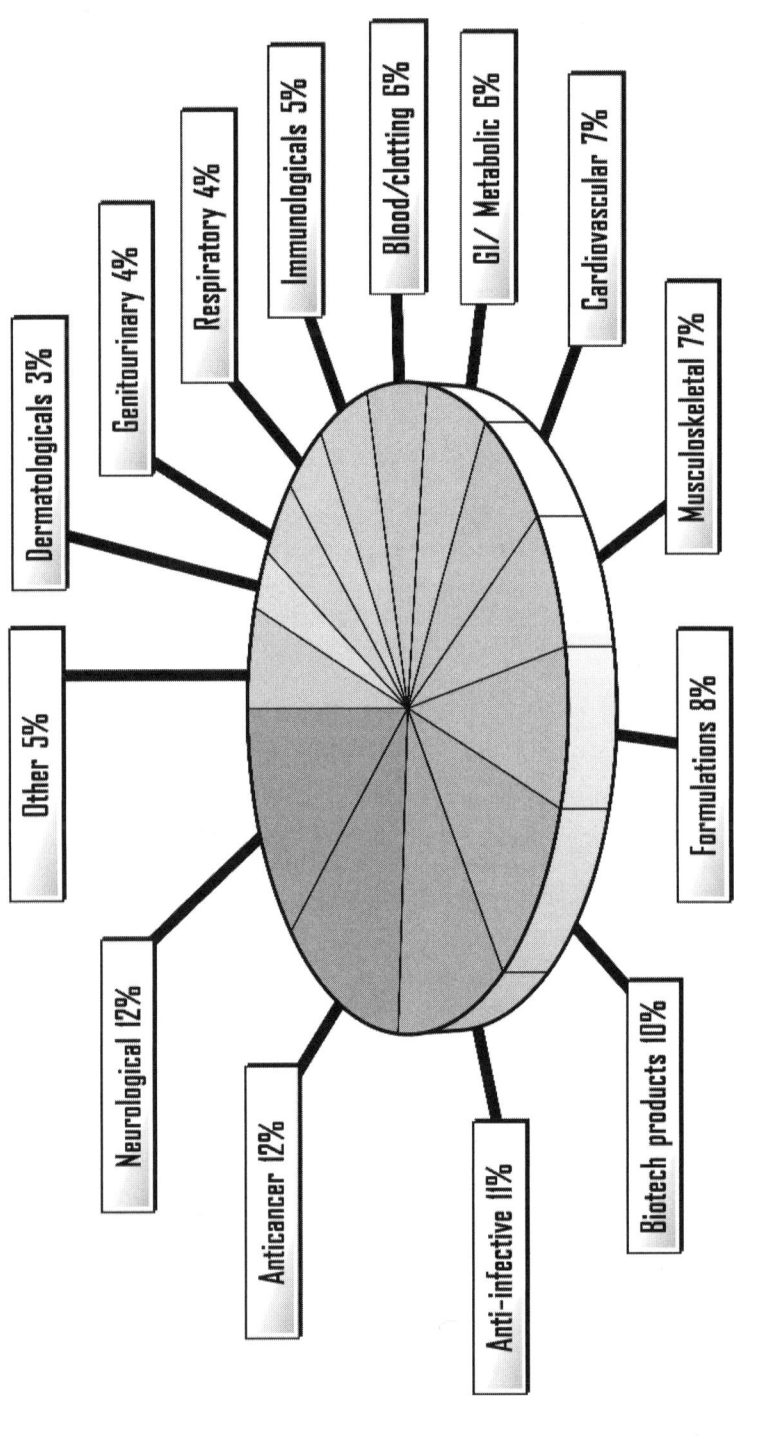

Figure 1.4. Therapeutic Distribution of NASs.

Drug Development and Industry Trends

1. Clinical endpoints for the disease should be well defined and measurable.
2. The NAS should be as effective, and ideally better, at treating the target disease than other candidates or marketed products.
3. The therapeutic index should be high (no observable adverse event level/ minimum effective dose).
4. The NAS should be chemically stable, in a clinically acceptable formulation, with production costs which allow retention of profit margin in a price-sensitive market.
5. The product should fulfill an unmet market need (eg previously untreatable population, reduced side effect profile, oral administration).
6. The patent life remaining after the projected licensing date will be sufficient to obtain an adequate Return On Investment (ROI).

Nevertheless, it is important not to delay rate-determining steps (eg construction of a pilot manufacturing plant) just because the next review milestone has not been reached (eg Phase IIb results not available). Thus a calculated risk is taken with such decisions, assuming success in other areas. This is justified by the financial loss of extending the critical path outweighing the advanced investment required to deliver on time.

INDUSTRY TRENDS

Demographic Market Expansion

Throughout the industrialized nations, the "baby boom" of the 1950s, coupled with major advances in healthcare have created an expansion in the elderly population, which is set to continue as life expectancies increase and birth rates fall.

By 2010 one-fifth of Italy's population will be over 65, causing a dramatic expansion of the healthcare market: 80% of an individual's lifetime healthcare costs are incurred after the age of 75. Strategic marketers in the pharmaceutical industry are following this trend with a resultant massive concentration of R&D effort towards the afflictions of this group: depression, dementia/Alzheimer's, Parkinson's, stroke, diabetes, osteoporosis, rheumatoid arthritis, breast cancer, melanoma, ischemic heart disease, incontinence, postural hypotension etc.

Windley reported that in 1998 the NASs in development were distributed by therapeutic category as shown in Figure 1.4.

Increasing Risk

The cost of developing new drugs is constantly and rapidly increasing. In 1987 the cost of bringing a NAS to market was approximately US$ 231 million. By

2001 this had risen to US$ 802 million (Tufts Center for the Study of Drug Development (Tufts CSDD)). Increasing demands from the world's regulatory agencies in recent years (eg ICH GCP Guidelines) means the acceleration of this trend both now and in future years.

The number of clinical studies required by the FDA for a NDA rose from 35 in 1988 to 65 in 1995. Studies are getting longer and more complex — the average number of procedures required by a protocol almost doubled from 100 to 190 in the period 1991–95. This is reflected in a similar rise since the mid-1980s in the cost per clinical study patient.

Although the potential for profit is increasing, so are the financial risks. It is estimated that for every one NAS launched on the market:

- 5–10,000 candidate molecules will be screened
- 250 will be evaluated in preclinical models
- 12 will enter Phase I clinical pharmacology
- Six will progress into Phase II clinical studies and two to three into Phase III.

The further the product progresses, the greater the financial commitment. The losses associated with failure in late Phase III can be devastating for a company (eg flosequinan, lexipafant).

Emphasis on NASs

In order to maximize ROI, the pharmaceutical strategy has shifted from "me too" products and line extensions, to the development of "blockbuster" NASs with added therapeutic value. The Tufts CSDD reported in 2002 that the top 10 percent of newly marketed drugs account for half the financial returns on all new drug development. This has focused attention on the new discovery approaches coming from the emergent biotechnology and genomics laboratories. The major pharmaceutical manufacturers now have licencing deals with, or have acquired, small biopharmaceuticals companies in order to maintain innovative R&D pipelines.

Market Consolidation

Pharmaceuticals manufacturers are seeking to minimize their risk by leveraging economies of scale. The late 1990s were characterized by a series of large-scale mergers and acquisitions between many of the major players: eg the formation of Astra Zeneca, Glaxo SmithKline, Pharmacia & Upjohn, Novartis, Sanofi Synthelabo, Celltech Chiroscience, and Aventis.

Drug Development and Industry Trends

Faster Synthesis and Screening

Increases in the length and number of clinical studies required for product registration have been largely offset by time savings at the discovery stage, through the use of combinatorial chemistry and high throughput screening. Advances in genomics have also allowed more precise targeting of receptor molecules. The expected lead-time for a NAS from discovery to market approval has thus remained stable through the 1990s at 11–13 years, depending on indication (CMR International).

Focus on Maximizing Patented Market Life

Time to market before patent expiry is now a major profitability issue for pharmaceuticals manufacturers. Kermani and Findlay estimated in 2002 that a globally marketed blockbuster NAS could expect to generate US$ 2.7 million in sales every day while patent-protected. In the first year off patent, 42% of Glaxo Wellcome's anti-ulcer drug ranitidine earnings were lost to generic competition.

The present effective patent term is 20 years, but more than half of this is consumed before the manufacturer can start to see any ROI.

The short patent protection period remaining at launch creates a need for simultaneous worldwide marketing. This is aided by an increasing trend towards international harmonization of regulatory standards (eg ICH GCP) and acceptance of regulatory approvals between national authorities (eg EU MRP).

E-Technology Applications

Since much of pharma R&D is about collecting, validating and analyzing information, the industry has benefited enormously from the e-revolution, and will continue to do so as manufacturers and regulatory agencies move towards paper-free drug development. Applications range from computer-assisted ligand-receptor modeling, through project tracking, centralized treatment randomization, and web-enabled data capture, to Computer-Assisted New Drug Application (CANDA) review. In Europe, the EMEA are currently rolling out an integrated safety database linked to a study register, which sponsors will be required to update electronically. The up-front investment required for the establishment of such systems is quickly justified by the profits generated by earlier product launch, and reduced R&D labor costs.

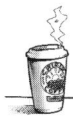

Chapter 2

Contract Research Organizations (CROs)

OUTSOURCING TO CROs

Since the mid 1980s cost pressures have driven the practice of outsourcing R&D activities, in order to cut the overhead risk of in-house/on-site R&D resourcing. This has lead to the emergence of a new corporate breed known as CROs. These companies specialize in providing one or more of: preclinical/toxicology, clinical development, analytical testing, biometrics and regulatory affairs/ quality assurance (QA) as services to pharma clients.

The primary manufacturer delegates some (or all) of its responsibilities as "sponsor" to the CRO, for the purpose of the development project. This enables sponsors to staff for the valleys rather than the peaks of the research cycle, thereby converting fixed costs into variable costs.

In many cases, geographic coverage, expertise and systems of CROs exceed those of the sponsor, and outsourcing then becomes a strategy for rapid globalized development and registration.

This had traditionally been associated with Phase III clinical development. More recently, the market has broadened to include discovery and preclinical services together with Phases I–II and health economics assessments, as pharma companies find value in outsourcing more and more of their R&D functions.

In 2002 Technomark reported that there are 167 clinical CROs with offices in Europe and 292 in the USA. Of the 25 leading companies, 18 are based in the US, three in Canada, two in the UK, one in Ireland and one in Germany.

The proportion of worldwide pharma/biotech R&D spending outsourced to CROs is expected to increase from 20% in 2001 to almost 30% in 2005, when the market will have doubled on its 1998 value to US$ 12.1 billion (Credit Suisse First Boston; Bear, Stearns & Co).

Economics

Clients are generally billed by CROs based on hourly rates for work done plus expenses. Utilization is typically 70–85%. The hourly rates include an overhead factor to cover non-project corporate costs. Overhead can vary from 15–50%, generally increasing with size of company.

Profit margins range from 8–14% with the overhead-burdened companies forced by competition to operate at the lower end of this range, relying on high volume programs to generate revenues. As a general rule, aggregating both billable and non-billable job classes, annual revenue generation in the CRO industry is US$ 88,000–97,000 per capita (Technomark). In 1999 Jones reported the professional billing rates of 14 leading CROs in the UK (Figure 2.1).

Job Title	UK £/hour		
	Low	Average	High
Physician	80	103	150
Project Manager	53	73	107
CRA/Monitor	39	51	61
CT Assistant	33	41	61
Data Manager	24	55	107
Statistician	44	61	94
Medical Writer	46	62	73

Figure 2.1. UK Billing Rates of 14 Leading CROs.

The major sponsors now have their own clinical study costing models, and are familiar with the billing rates or unit activity prices of the top tier CROs. Using market influence to drive down CRO profit margins, once a fashionable activity, has now been abandoned by experienced sponsors as being a self-defeating approach long term. They are now more interested working with a CRO who can add fiscal value to their drug in terms of time to market. Selection is thus based on possession of systems and procedures which will deliver a product acceptable to regulatory agencies worldwide earlier than other bidders. A CRO with healthy profits to invest is far more likely to provide this.

Quality

Prior to the introduction of the ICH GCP guidelines quality was an added value differentiator within the CRO market. Sponsors now expect this as an industry standard however, and will not consider companies that do not have formalized internal QA programs for pivotal research contracts.

Capabilities

Sponsors speak of outsourcing as being the process of finding the best fit between the needs of a project and the strengths of a CRO. The CRO should be seen to have available human resources suitably experienced to conduct the work, therapeutic area expertise within the management team and a stable workforce. Secondly, these resources should be able to operate across the geographic regions required. This usually means native-speaking Clinical Research Associates (CRAs), and regulatory affairs experience in the territory concerned, ideally operating from a local office.

As dictated by the nature of the study, particular technologies (eg project or data management systems) or facilities (eg central laboratory, drug packaging/distribution,QA auditors) may offer advantages to the sponsor.

Increasingly, outsourcing managers will also make corporate financial risk assessments of the CRO before entering into a partnership.

In terms of size, the larger the CRO, the greater the range of services and geographic coverage it can provide. There is a place, however, for smaller CROs who concentrate on a limited range of niche services or therapeutic expertise, and can offer lower billing rates. Technomark estimates that the top 20 CROs account for 58% of the total market. Most of these have annual revenues in excess of US$ 50 million, making them comparable to or larger than the R&D departments of their clients. Nevertheless it is notable that between 2000–2001 revenues for the top five CROs grew by only 8.5% compared with 22.8% for the remaining 15. This suggests that sponsors are preferring to work with medium-sized CROs instead of their bigger brothers.

Personal Chemistry

Many sponsors cite the personal qualities of the CRO project manager and their interactions with his/her team as being the most important factor in determining the success of a project. They expect to meet the potential project manager prior to awarding the contract, and thus this has become a decision criterion.

Long-Term Partnerships

As the financial value to sponsors of outsourcing to minimize product development risk has increased, so their strategists have begun building CROs into their long range planning, rather than calling on them as emergency services in the last resort.

It then became immediately recognized that the most efficient partnerships would involve trust, shared risk and harmonization of systems and procedures. Thus the late 1990s saw the creation of a new industry job title: CRO manager. The logical extension of this is, having invested in integrating a CRO almost as part of the sponsor company, further efficiencies and synergies follow if the relationship is continued on to further projects. Here, the sponsor is at the level of sharing its PDPs at an early stage in order that the CRO can staff ahead appropriately to meet the expected demand. Study lead times are reduced and financial and scope of work issues dealt with quickly within the framework of a master consulting agreement.

Sponsors are not blind to the pitfalls of committing completely to one CRO however (CRO failure, loss of quality, price creep); and the exclusive provider agreements signed in the early 1990s have been largely replaced by panels of three to four preferred vendors.

The Contracting Process

From advertising, analyst and personal sources, the sponsor will draw up a first-list of CROs who appear to have the right mix of capabilities and services. These will be invited to sign a confidentiality agreement, and make general presentations to the sponsor. Many sponsors then ask each candidate to follow up by completing a standardized CRO Evaluation Questionnaire.

The sponsor will then select a short list of three to four CROs, who will formally be asked to present a time and cost proposal as a bid for contract. This will take the form of a Request For Proposal (RFP) document, which should clearly define the trial design, timeline, delegated responsibilities, and scope of work. It is imperative that each CRO receives an identical RFP, so that all bidders are working from the same page.

The CRO representative then asks the internal clinical team to provide information on how and where the sponsor's project could be conducted, and highlight any problems or added value opportunities. This generally involves canvassing potential investigators and opinion leaders. The feasibility assessment ideally should be able to provide all the assumptions needed for costing the project (number of patients, recruitment rates, treatment period, number of sites, etc.).

Working with input from the clinical team, the CRO representative then prepares a proposal document. The time available for this is generally 10 working days. A project manager will generally be nominated at this stage, and will attend subsequent sponsor meetings.

If the bid is successful, the sponsor will issue a Letter of Intent to Proceed to

Contract (LOI). This agrees to cover the CRO's fees and expenses for the work as defined in the proposal, until a legal contractual agreement is signed. No project work or financial commitments should be undertaken by the CRO until such a letter is received.

The final contractual agreement may take 3–5 months to negotiate, during which time the project will be set up and running, though the operational and budget components will generally be unchanged from the original proposal. If there have been previous collaborations between the parties, the process may be streamlined by add-on to an existing contractual agreement.

Throughout the life of a project the CRO account manager keeps in contact with the sponsor and internal project manager in order to first troubleshoot potential budget, contractual, and customer satisfaction issues and second, to identify and develop further business opportunities.

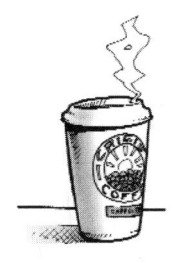

Chapter 3

The Role of the Clinical Study Project Manager

THE PROJECT TEAM

The day-to-day running of a clinical study requires the coordinated input from the following specialist groups (see Figure 3.1):

Biostatistics: Statistical Analysis Plan (SAP), study design, randomisation schedule; data tables and listings, difference testing

Study production: Study drug manufacture, packaging, distribution, randomisation

Clinical monitoring: Investigator selection, training, site management, monitoring

Central laboratory: Shipment, analysis, reporting of biological specimens

Pharmacovigilance: Serious Adverse Event (SAE) reporting and quality control (QC)

Data management: Case Report/Record Form (CRF), database/edit check design, data entry and QC

Medical writing: Protocol, clinical study report

Other departments which will contribute to the study on an as-needed basis are:

- regulatory affairs
- QA
- manufacturing
- marketing
- preclinical development
- drug discovery
- medical communications
- finance

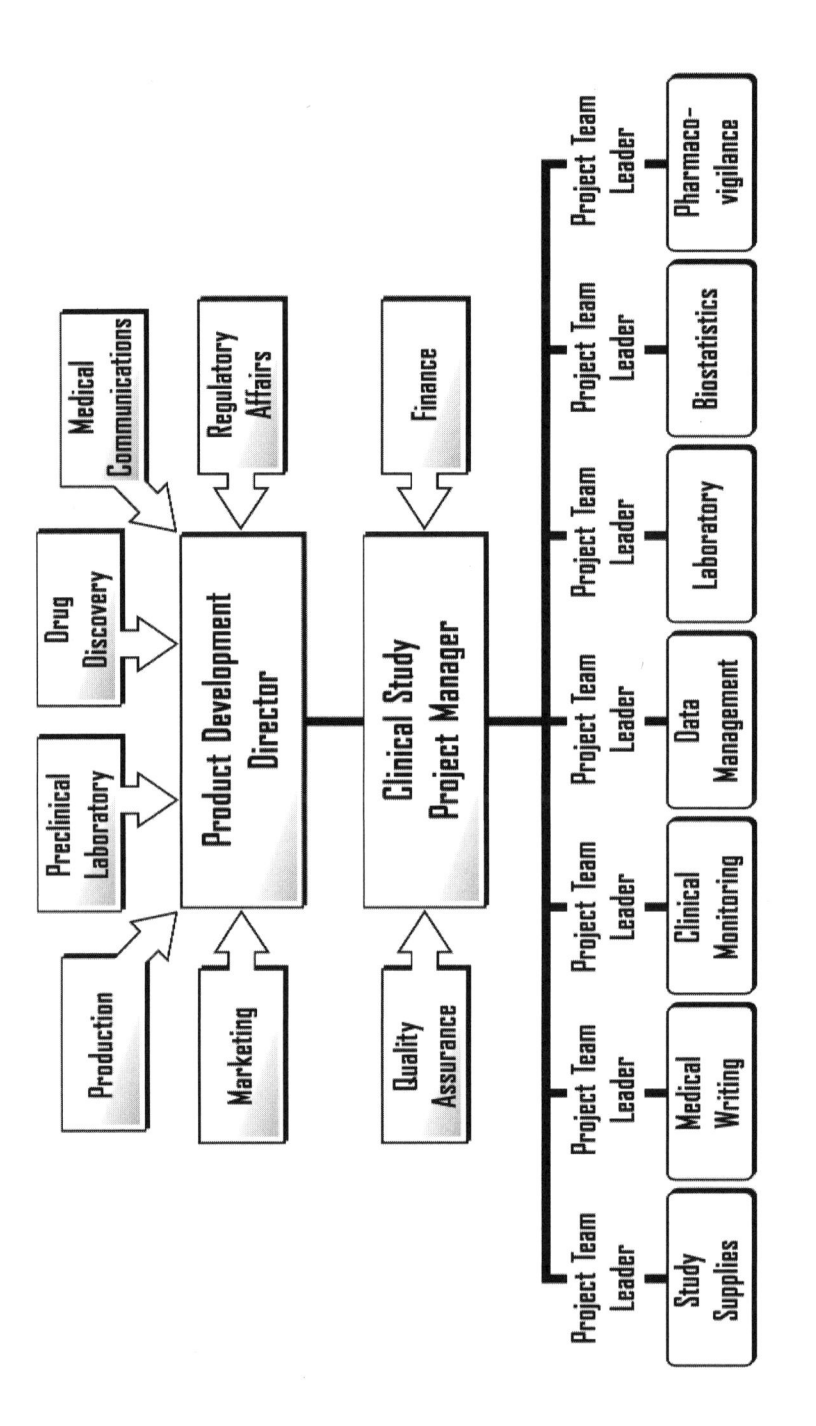

Figure 3.1. Clincal Study Project Team.

Matrix Management

The project activities of staff reporting to you will be your responsibility. They are your team, and will look to you for direction. Nevertheless, it will commonly be the case that they have separate line managers, drawn from their own specialities. Indeed they will typically be also working for other project managers in parallel. This is known as matrix management, and in its simplest follows the scheme shown over (Figure 3.2).

This is undoubtedly a sensible and flexible approach to resourcing projects. It allows staff to be allocated as needed in response to changing project demands. As such it is particularly suited to the cyclical nature of clinical research.

Nevertheless, the matrix requires careful consideration to avoid conflicts of interest. In an ideal world, Projects A and B have balanced resource demands (ie peaks match valleys). However, add in Project C and things start to get a little strained, particularly if the timeline for A slips so as to clash with a busy spell on B, and a team member gets sick. Here it is the responsibility of the relevant project managers to agree a solution with the line manager(s).

Team Dynamics

For a project team to be productive and effective, the following dynamics are necessary:

- The membership represents an adequate staffing at the appropriate skill levels
- There is a relaxed atmosphere in which people feel committed and motivated
- Overall objectives are understood and agreed to (buy in)
- Goal-directed discussions in which all members participate
- Team members share information freely and listen to each other
- Open expression of disagreement is accepted
- Decisions are reached by consensus
- Criticism/ reassessment is frequent but constructive
- People are free to express ideas
- Each team member takes responsibility for his/her deliverables
- Control and influence is balanced to the team structure
- Individuals are adaptable and flexible to changes in project requirements

At its peak, a Phase III study may have 50 project team members working together. Psychologists tell us that the magic number for an effective group is seven players. A large team thus needs to be cut into bite-sized chunks. There are many ways to do this. In Figure 3.1 I have shown the functional groups working together under seven team leaders, who then act as a management

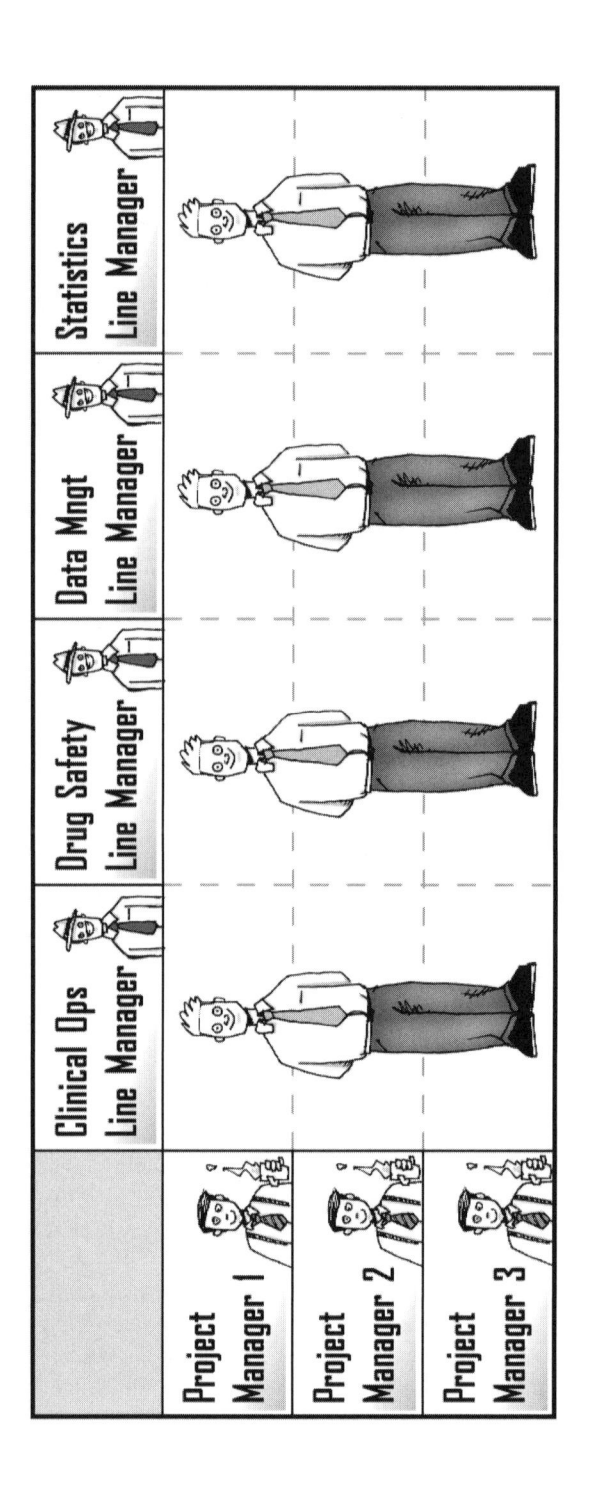

Figure 3.2. Matrix Management Structure.

group themselves. Alternatives are geographic teams, or the establishment of small cross-functional work groups dedicated to particular tasks.

THE FUNCTION OF THE MANAGER

As mentioned earlier, the operational activities which combine to make a study are highly specialized. This means that project managers are unlikely to have detailed experience or knowledge of all areas. They thus rely on judgement and technical advice from their team specialists. Many use the analogy of a soccer coach who is vital to winning, but is neither goalkeeper, defender nor striker. I prefer the idea of a catalyst, which brings together molecules in a way which makes them react. The catalyst is not a part of the reaction, merely the facilitator. When people ask me what I do, I tell them: "I don't do anything; and if I did, I wouldn't be doing my job."

What project managers do have to do, however, is take directional decisions for the good of the study. They need the authority to engage all managerial and technical resources required to complete the project successfully. Within this they uniquely have ultimate responsibility for quality, timeline and budget.

Specifically, a project manager is empowered to take the following actions:

- Act as the focus of study communications
- Establish a plan to achieve the goals
- Ensure adequate staffing, training and resourcing
- Resolve matrix management issues with line managers
- Track actual progress against planned achievements
- Take major steering decisions
- Control the allocation and expenditure of budget
- Provide leadership to and maintain the focus of the team members
- Resolve conflicting priorities and cross-disciplinary challenges

From the role described it can be seen that the following personal characteristics are desirable in a project manager:

- Ability to delegate
- Good communication skills
- Knowledge of company
- Understanding of matrix management
- Decision-making ability
- Enthusiasm, energy, assertiveness
- Versatility, flexibility
- Ability to deal with risk and uncertainty
- Honesty and integrity

- Experience in clinical studies
- Creative problem solving

Nevertheless if you put in a lonely hearts ad for someone with all of the above, you might be disappointed with the result. Given the diversity of "folks," different individuals will have variable strengths and weaknesses, which combine to produce their own management style. Personally I find myself to be a shape-shifter who moves between all of Meredith Belbin's personality types during the course of a project.

Decision Making

Having identified decision making as one of the key activities of a project manager, it is worth examining how decisions are made.

The first step is to define the issue. You must clarify the scope of the question to be answered or problem to be resolved. Clinical studies are multi-factorial jigsaws however, and this is not always a straightforward exercise in itself.

A useful technique is to analyze and reduce the subject into key components. You may find that a particular issue is a combination of questions requiring separate decisions. It is often the case that a complex problem can be successfully dealt with by breaking it down into a series of simple solutions. This may then throw into sharp relief one central issue on which attention must be focused.

Once a horse race is won, everyone can tell you the outcome. Most can pick a favorite by the half-way post. Seasoned punters will study previous form and place their bets before the race. The point is that the more information you have, the easier it is to make the right decision. However, just as bookie will give you better odds before the race day, the earlier a project manager makes a decision, the greater its value.

The mark of a good project manager is the ability to make the right call based on limited information. How is this done? Well it may be that previous experience of a similar situation allows accurate prediction of current events. The project manager may also know that the outcome will be ultimately driven by one or two factors, and base the decision on that information. When planning how many burgers to buy for a barbeque party, I have learned to look not at the guest list, but at the weather forecast.

Indeed it will normally be the case that not all the required information is available. The trap here is to delay decision making until everything is known. The skilled decision-maker will initiate gathering of critical information only (sub-decision) and act once that is received. A common compromise is to take the initial decision to go, but build in a review point (stop/continue) which coincides with the new data becoming available.

Judging Risk

Every decision carries with it a risk. The risk is the negative consequence of the unintended outcome occurring. I was once leading a group of children in mountains when a dense fog appeared. We came to a point where we could either travel several extra miles on a path we could see, or follow a shorter route blind across broken ground. The short route passed by steep cliffs, and in the fog I could not guarantee we would see them if we strayed from the compass bearing. Here the risk of failure was lethal, and I weighted the decision to take the long way home.

While every endeavor should be made to "do the right thing," analysis should be made of the cost of other outcomes. In some cases the cost of failure may be acceptable when compared to the benefit of an early decision. It may also be possible to take actions which reduce the cost of negative results (eg including additional doses to study design), thereby adjusting the balance in favor of benefits.

Judgement should also be made of the likelihood of success/failure. You should take any opportunity available to reduce the likelihood of a negative outcome (eg blood shipment temperature control) and thus create your own luck.

Last, but by no means least, you should take action. Having decided on a course to be followed, the necessary instructions and resourcing should be given for its implementation.

HIGH-RISE VS HANDS-OFF

The medieval feudal system can still be seen today in many corporate management structures. Chain mail armor may have been replaced by suits, but the tell-tale signs are a pyramidal hierarchy with one all-powerful leader issuing commands from the top.

I liken this formation to a high-rise tower block. Indeed it is often the case that seniority within such an organization is measured by which floor of the building you get off the elevator. With high-rise management, a piece of new information enters the lobby at street level, and like a hapless delivery boy is forced to tour each floor in succession before it can finally be decided upon at the top. This is not the end of the story however, because the resulting command then has to laboriously retrace the entry route before it can find the operative at the front desk who will take action.

Thus there is an organizational inertia which slows responsiveness. In addition, the successive management tiers build in a rigidity which makes changing focus or direction problematic for the organization.

In the fast-moving, high-risk pharma business environment, high-rise management is becoming increasingly less appropriate. The industry is now moving towards a more "hands-off" or decentralized approach. Here decision-making authority is vested at the lowest possible level, in order to maximize responsiveness and flexibility. Information technology is used to maintain a corporate awareness of what is going on, but it is the staff on the ground floor who are in the driving seat.

The result is a flat corporate world, but one which can continually adapt to changing regulatory, scientific, project, market and commercial needs. The hands-off approach of course relies on good staff training, a topic covered in Chapter 10. It also encourages horizontal rather that vertical interactions between functions (eg data management, biostatistics) and thus is a good fit with matrix management.

Delegation

Nevertheless, drawing flat "hands-off" organograms is worthless if there is no effective delegation from the Project Manager. Delegation is the art of assigning decision-making authority to other members of the team. This is the foundation of decentralized project management, and can be broken into five steps:

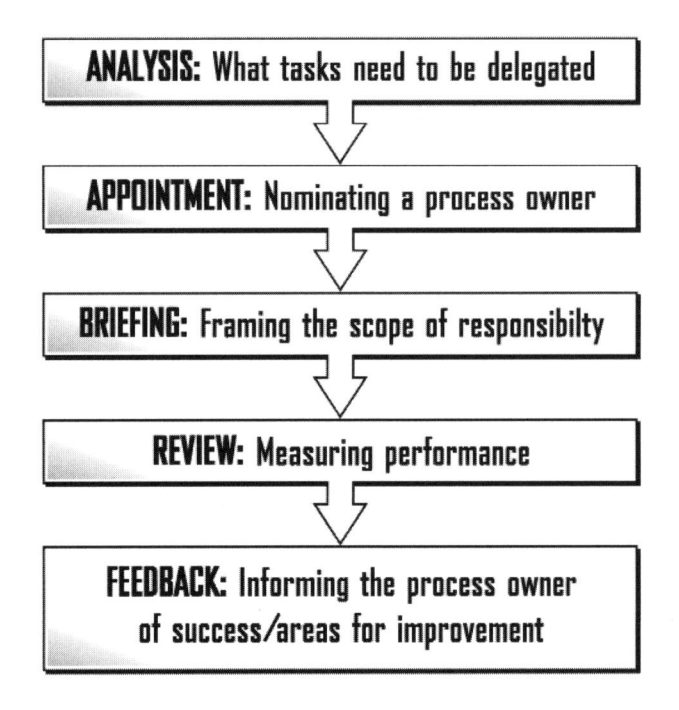

```
ANALYSIS: What tasks need to be delegated
              ↓
APPOINTMENT: Nominating a process owner
              ↓
BRIEFING: Framing the scope of responsibilty
              ↓
REVIEW: Measuring performance
              ↓
FEEDBACK: Informing the process owner
          of success/areas for improvement
```

Figure 3.3. The Delegation Process.

Role of the Clinical Study Project Manager

You should feel comfortable to delegate:

- Activities which come within the scope of an individual's job description
- Problems or activities which require detailed technical exploration and analysis
- Tasks which will positively develop the skills of an individual in contributing to the project, and their career growth
- Activities which are more cost effectively performed at a lower level
- Tasks which are not specific to the project manager or have been directly assigned to you

Pitfalls to be avoided

- You nominate a process owner, but then continually interfere or micromanage.
- The process owner exceeds or does not meet their responsibility because the scope of work was not clearly defined.
- You overload an inexperienced/inappropriately qualified person because of a staffing deficiency.

You don't delegate because you fear that:

- Your staff isn't up to the job
- You can do it faster yourself
- You think people will see this as dumping on others

You delegate because:

- The task is too difficult for you
- You want to shift responsibility away from yourself

Staff who are not used to hands-off management may initially find this unsettling. They will return repeatedly, asking for instruction. They should be progressively encouraged to run further with the ball before reporting back. As mutual trust grows, then more decisions and activities can be assigned. If a team member does make a mistake however, you must be prepared to take the blame yourself (the buck stops with you). Nevertheless, you should then work more closely with the individual concerned, to help them improve their decision making skills.

In addition to creating an organization which is more flexible and responsive to changes, there are several spin-offs from taking your hands off the wheel. First, team motivation will increase, as members become stakeholders in the decisions made. Second, fresh ideas coming from staff with different backgrounds will enrich the capabilities of the team. Last, you will spend less time on operational functions, and more on what you should really be doing: managing.

Chapter 4

Goals and Standards

OBJECTIVES AND MILESTONES

Before setting out onto the high seas, every captain needs to know his port of destination in order to chart a course. Similarly every company will have a mission statement which defines its ambitions. For a large multinational, this may at the broadest level be to maximize shareholder ROI. The remit of the pharmaceutical division may be more specific, in that its contribution would be perhaps to launch one blockbuster NAS every five years.

The planning of activities requires three elements. First, the target or desired outcome (**goal**), second, the framework of responsibilities and quality standards within which this is to be achieved (**benchmarking**), and third, the route to be taken (**method**).

Goal

For a drug development program, the goal will be to produce a safe and effective new medicine which has a commercial advantage in the marketplace, and that can be rapidly licensed worldwide in order to maximize ROI for the duration of its patented life. As discussed in Chapter 1, the strategies may be to focus on diseases which are poorly controlled by conventional treatments, to exploit new technologies, medical discoveries, or work in therapeutic areas which are expanding (eg age-related diseases).

Benchmarking

The benchmarking is to all intents and purposes defined by the legal demands of national drug regulatory authorities. Separate examination of this is made in the following section.

Method

As to the method, a multi-disciplinary team will be established at the concept stage for the strategic planning of the product specification, disease markets and potential revenues. The team will then receive input from the marketing, medical, drug discovery, production, regulatory affairs, preclinical and clinical development groups. A Product Development Plan will then be devised to meet the regulatory, production, medical and commercial needs of the project.

A key theme in the structuring of the PDP is that like a Russian doll there should be cascading tiers of objectives. Thus at each level of magnification it can be seen what every department, team, group, or individual has to deliver in order to make the study a success.

In addition to possessing successive horizontal levels of detail, the PDP should also contain on its time axis interim objectives, or milestones. Milestones are short-term targets, tailored for each group to aim for. They have a useful motivational role, especially if the final deliverable is over a year away. Additionally, progress in achieving each milestone can be used to track the project status (see Chapter 8).

The most effective way to prepare a PDP is to ask the process-owners themselves. The hands-off project manager recognizes that these are the people best placed to optimize the work practices within their area. Here the role of the project manager is thus limited to assembling the pieces of the plan provided by the functional teams. This also has the benefit of fostering an environment where team members feel that they are stakeholders in the overall grand design.

CLINICAL RESEARCH STANDARDS

As mentioned earlier, the benchmarking for drug development comes largely from international guidelines and national legislation. Following the medical abuse of prisoners in Nazi concentration camps during the Second World War, the 1947 Nuremberg Code sought to establish a bill of rights for subjects participating in clinical experiments. This for the first time introduced the concept of informed consent. In 1964 the World Medical Association (WMA) extended these principles in an international declaration made at their Helsinki assembly. The so-called Declaration of Helsinki, now in its fifth revision, is today the accepted keystone of ethical standards in biomedical research.

Many elements from the Declaration of Helsinki were evident in the Title 21 Code of Federal Regulations Part 312 introduced in 1977 by the US Government with the IND-NDA system. This then became the regulatory model followed to a greater or lesser extent by other industrialized nations. Following the publishing of GCP Guidelines by the European Community CPMP in 1991 however, a plan of international convergence was begun with the establishment of the International Conference on Harmonization. The objective was to create between the US, EU and Japan a common set of regulations governing the design, conduct, recording and reporting of clinical studies. In this it borrowed the "best bits" from the EU, FDA, Nordic, Canadian, Australian and World Health Organization (WHO) guidelines.

Goals and Standards

The result was the ICH Step 4 Tripartite Guideline on GCP, May 1996 which is now being integrated into the legal systems of the signatories. In structure it identifies three areas of responsibility: the IRB, investigator and sponsor; and lists the documents and records which are regarded essential to the study management.

IRB

The IRB is described as an independent committee concerned with reviewing the ethical aspects of proposed clinical studies. GCP lists its responsibilities in safeguarding the rights, safety and well-being of subjects; the documents to be assessed; required constitution; and the procedures for exercising its governing role in the local approval of study applications.

Investigator

The term investigator is used for the research physician responsible for clinical management of a subject in a study, dispensing of study drug, and collection of data. Once again GCP defines the obligations of this individual, and sets out the activities required in their conduct of the experiment. Particular reference is made to the investigator and his/her staff having the appropriate qualifications, training, time, equipment and facilities to perform study in compliance with the protocol, and manage the investigational product. There is discussion not only of the investigator's duty of medical care to the subject, but also detail on how informed consent should be obtained. It is also notable that while in practice it is the sponsor who communicates with the IRB and prepares study reports, in GCP these roles are assigned to the investigator.

Sponsor

In GCP, a sponsor is the organization managing and financing the study, which is also usually the drug manufacturer. The following areas of responsibility are listed, together with the activities required:

- QA and QC
- Relevant medical expertise
- Trial management
- Data handling
- Record keeping
- Investigator selection
- Allocation of responsibilities

Protocol

There is nothing new about preparing a protocol to plan out the objectives, design, methods, statistics and organization of a clinical study. Nevertheless, GCP now provides a unified definition of the topics to be covered and structure for this, as indicated below.

- General information
- Background information
- Objectives and purpose
- Trial design
- Selection and withdrawal of subjects
- Treatment of subjects
- Assessment of efficacy
- Assessment of safety
- Statistics
- Direct access to source data
- QC and QA
- Ethics
- Data handling
- Financing and insurance
- Publication policy
- Supplements

Protocol design is discussed further in the next section.

Investigator's Brochure

A fundamental of GCP is that research subjects, investigators and IRBs should have access to the latest available pharmaceutical, toxicity, pharmacology and clinical data on the test medication(s). This is to allow informed decision to be made on medical risks and benefits before and during the study. Much of this information is provided by means of an investigator's brochure. In the case of research subjects, summarized statements from this are in turn used to prepare the subject information forms, which underpin the informed consent process. GCP defines the purpose, distribution, format and required contents of an investigator's brochure (IB).

Essential Documents

Finally GCP provides an archiving plan such that an unequivocal audit trail is

Goals and Standards

left at every level of study management. My spin on this is that if the crew of the *Marie Celeste* had been following GCP, then we would know what had happened to them. A list of documents deemed as "essential" are presented in an elegant table that shows their purpose, filing location and the stage of the project at which they are required. In general terms, this necessitates local Investigator Study Files (ISFs), and a centralized Sponsor Trial Master File (TMF).

WRITING A STUDY PROTOCOL

ICH GCP defines a study protocol as the document which "...*describes the objectives, design, methodology, statistical considerations, and organisation of a trial.*" As well as being a plan of the project goals and quality standards, it also functions as an operational manual for the daily conduct of the experiment. Just as an architect's blueprint will unify the activities of bricklayers, carpenters, electricians, plasterers and plumbers to build a house, the protocol will specify how different functions within the project team interact to complete the study.

The intended readership will include investigators, study nurses, pharmacists, technicians, CRAs, project management, data management, medical writing, regulatory affairs, production supplies support, pharmacovigilance, regulatory authority reviewers, IRB members, and QA auditors.

Responsibility for preparation of the protocol, however, falls to the project manager, and will be one of your first activities. GCP provides the list of contents, and it is likely that there will be company standards for the generic text. Nevertheless, to "join the dots," you will require specialist input from the project physician, principal investigator, statistician, study production support, regulatory affairs; and access to the latest pharmaceutical, toxicity, pharmacology, and clinical data on the test medication (ie investigator's brochure).

You may decide to compile the document yourself, or delegate this to a medical writer and adopt a purely editorial role. Whoever is involved, there will be an enormous pressure to complete the task as early as possible, since it is the mother of all critical activities. Nevertheless, in the shifting world of drug development, not all the pieces of the jigsaw may be available. The final number of investigators required may not be known, some long-term animal studies may not yet be complete, there may be a late change in the product formula, investigators may differ on the classification of a disease or an at-risk population, rating scales and available treatments may vary between countries. A decision will then have to be taken to proceed with a document which is the best fit between current knowledge and the urgency to publish.

While it generally should not take more than 10 working days to collate a draft protocol, gaining final agreement from all the stakeholders and QC reviewers often takes considerably longer. Once this has been achieved there is then a rush to submit to regulatory agencies and IRBs. These bodies often request changes to the protocol however, and it is not uncommon to be forced into amending the protocol prior to the start of the study. A second submission of the study is then required, which delays start-up. This is a clear case of more haste, less speed. The way of squaring this circle is to have early review of the draft protocol by a wide panel of company regulatory specialists and opinion leader physicians from the planned countries. This may add a week or two to the initial task, but has the potential to save months in the long run.

The following is a gardener's guide to protocol writing, in which I have summarized the main topics that need to be covered, and shown where they sit in the document.

1. General Information

The front page of the document should show the study title, protocol code number, and version date for identification purposes. It is recommended that the protocol number and version date also appear as footers on every page throughout.

Second, there should be identification with addresses and contact details of the sponsor, investigator(s), laboratory, or any CRO with responsibilities in the study management.

This should be followed by a section for stakeholders from these organizations to sign agreement to comply with the protocol and principles of GCP.

2. Background Information

The first half of the background information section will be drawn from the summary of the investigator's brochure. Far from being a lazy short-cut, electronic copying and pasting of this text word-for-word has the advantage of accuracy, and avoids delays in re-checking (QC) the information. Topics which should be covered are the test product chemistry and pharmacy, preclinical data, and any previous clinical data.

Next, a rationale should be developed showing how the information collected to date justifies the proposed study design and target population. The section should then close with a statement that ICH GCP will be followed in all aspects of the study management.

3. Objectives and Purpose

Section 3 should clarify in concrete terms what the primary and secondary objectives are for performing the study, and demonstrate why gathering such information is necessary.

Goals and Standards

4. Study Design

In describing the study design, you should begin by showing the experimental approach which has been selected (eg crossover, group-comparative, double-blind, etc). There should be mention of the clinical endpoints which will be used, and clear definition of the stages and duration of the study (eg run-in, treatment, follow-up). It is then a good idea to show visually how the planned procedures lie vs time, by drawing a flow-chart. You should also document how the various treatment groups will be organized, and how many subjects will be recruited to each. Lastly you are required to make a statement on the number of investigational centers and the rate of patient enrollment. I would advise keeping this as vague as possible, to give yourself operational flexibility. I normally say something like: "Based on an expected recruitment rate of one patient/center/month, it is envisaged that it will take 30 investigators one year to complete the study, although this may be subject to change."

5. Selection and Withdrawal

This is the most thumbed chapter, and also the subject of greatest debate. It is where the entry criteria are listed that define the population sample. These should be divided into inclusion criteria, which are the target demographics and disease characteristics; and exclusion criteria, which are undesirable factors which would either place subjects at undue risk or bias the results. These items should be very carefully worded, following unambiguous medical terminology, and using standardized definitions (eg rating scale scores, diagnostic test values, clinical chemistry units, etc). It is important to note however that the contents of the entry criteria will directly influence the eventual licensed product labeling. Thus exclusion of particular age groups, forms or severity of disease could, in the absence of other data, later prevent prescribing to those sufferers.

As well as providing rules for entering the study, this section should explain from the outset how protocol violations will be managed, and to what degree these will be tolerated. Linked to this, there should be a description of the conditions under which subjects will be prematurely removed from the study. In addition to protocol violations, this should consider safety issues, and the patient's right to withdraw spontaneously. Whatever the reason, there should be a written procedure for performing a final clinical follow-up, and recording the reason for withdrawal.

Lastly there should be listed the conditions under which the study itself will be terminated. These will largely be: successful completion, discovery of an undue risk/lack of benefit, protocol non-compliance, or commercial/financial grounds.

6. Treatment

This is the section in which there will be pharmaceutical descriptions of all the formulations to be administered, together with the dose regimens required. There should also be explanation of how the study drug will be packaged, and examples of the labeling to be used.

It is important that the required storage conditions are specified. With regard to shelf life however, I would not advocate quoting an expiration date in the protocol, for the reasons discussed in Chapter 7. Nevertheless you could add a statement that chemical stability will be reconfirmed at regular (eg three-month) intervals.

There should however be detail on how treatments will be assigned to subjects, accounted for, and any randomization or stratification schemes. Blinding systems need to be explained, with a description of the procedure to be followed for emergency unblinding of a treatment.

7. Efficacy Assessments

The measurement of efficacy will be one of the primary objectives of the study. The parameters assessed will be specific to the disease and may require specialist technicians or equipment. Nevertheless, it is often the case that definitions of disease endpoints vary between nations, and you should take advice on which measurements will be accepted by the intended regulatory authorities.

Having selected a parameter on which to base the test of efficacy, the assessment method should be clearly set out in the protocol, together with the units of measurement, and timings of the evaluations. For more sophisticated procedures, it may also be appropriate to specify equipment calibration and QA procedures.

8. Safety Assessments

Safety is determined in a more generic fashion. The standard panel of tests would be a general physical examination, vital signs, ECG, haematology, biochemistry and urinalysis. As a minimum these should be measured prior to the administration of study drug to identify any at-risk subjects, and act as a baseline for future on-treatment test results. Additional safety parameters may be indicated by disease or drug class. Follow-up safety assessments should then be made at key points in the study, such as dose titrations and the post-treatment visit.

The second area of safety data collection is the recording of spontaneous adverse events. Here you should place the ICH GCP definitions of adverse events, and the criteria for serious or unexpected adverse events. The procedures and investigator obligations for reporting these should be detailed, together with the relevant pharmacovigilance contact numbers. In addition, there should be guidance on rating both event severity, and causal relationship to the test medication.

9. Visit Procedures

There is nothing in ICH GCP which says you have to include a visit task guide in a protocol. I have learned however that this is welcomed by study staff when present, and that mistakes (ie protocol violations) occur when it is not. I now always write a step-by-step list of what to do or tell the patient to do at each visit. This becomes particularly helpful as an *aide memoir* when instructions have to be given to the patient before the visit (eg complete diary card, withhold caffeine, etc), Interactive Voice Response System (IVRS) randomization codes have to be obtained, X-rays booked, or drug dispensed in advance.

10. Statistics

A key principle in scientific research is that the assay system for testing a hypothesis is established before the data are collected. Thus a fair trial is given, avoiding "fitting the test to the results." This goes for clinical studies too, and is integral to the protocol. The statistical analysis plan should be mapped out, stating the parameters which will be examined, and specifying the time-points which will be used for comparison (eg mean change in seated diastolic blood pressure at baseline vs after eight weeks treatment, compared between placebo and treatment groups). This will typically be both the primary efficacy, and safety end-points.

There should be reference to the method of hypothesis testing which will be employed (eg Analysis of Variance, chi-squared, Wilcoxon-Mann-Whitney etc), together with the level of statistical significance at which this will be determined. Linked to this, the statistician should show a justification for selection of the sample population (ie how many subjects), with assumptions of response size and variability.

In recognition that protocol violations will bias some of the data, there needs also to be in this section a set of minimum criteria for subject data to be included in the experimental analysis (per protocol evaluability). It should also be clear how bad data will be reported. This generally produces two data sets, an Intention-To-Treat (ITT) analysis, which includes all subjects enrolled, and the more exclusive per protocol group.

11. Direct Access

ICH GCP requires that there is a statement in the protocol in which the investigator allows representatives from regulatory authorities, the IRB and sponsor to directly inspect subject source data relevant to the study, for verification and QA audit purposes. I suggest you paraphrase the relevant sections from pages 4 and 20 of the guideline. In days gone by, this was a contentious issue of patient privacy in some health systems. However he enactment of GCP into local legislation has now largely resolved this.

12. Quality Control and Assurance

The quality section should open with a reference to which set of Standard Operating Procedures (SOPs) will be followed, with any exceptions. Typically these will be those of the sponsor, but this may vary if CROs and other contractors are participating.

Using GCP terminology, you then need to explain how QC of the data on site will operate. This will generally be periodic visits by CRAs in order to perform source data verification.

Continuing the theme, you should follow with an account of the in-house data cleaning process (double data comparison, automated edit checks, clinical review, query resolution), and how an error-free database is subsequently locked.

Lastly there should be generic reference to investigators being subject to randomly selected audit by specialist third party QA inspectors (ie sponsor, CRO, Regulatory Authority, IRB).

13. Ethics

The research ethics section is one where careful wording can save an IRB delay. This begins with an undertaking that the study will not be started by the investigator until IRB approval has been received. Similarly, you should also commit to submit any subsequent protocol amendments for review.

Second, there should be a detailed account of how informed consent will be obtained, and a brief summary of the contents of the Patient Information and Consent Form (PICF).

A procedure should be given for informing the family doctor of the subjects' participation in the study.

This is also the place for a statement on the intention to maintain subject anonymity in the data collected off-site; identification being limited to initials and study code number.

14. Data Handling

The data handling section is best written by your data management representative. It will outline the scheme by which information is recorded by the investigator (eg CRF), transferred in-house (eg fax), entered into the database, and archived.

There also needs to be mention of how other essential regulatory documents will additionally be retained in the TMF.

15. Finance and Insurance

This section should use standardized wording which demonstrates an intention to comply with ICH GCP on the issues of investigator costs, patient expenses, patient insurance, and investigator indemnification. Once again I would urge against locking yourself into specifics, since changing for example the investigator grant would then necessitate a protocol amendment. A point to note is that in Europe patient insurance and investigator indemnification are separate issues/activities, while in the US they are combined.

16. Publication Policy

While secrecy may have been covered by a separate confidential disclosure agreement, there will need to be publication of results at some stage. How this is to be managed should be described in the protocol. This is of particular interest for the investigators because for many, authorship of manuscripts is their motivation for participation. You should thus define the conditions for public release of data, listing any sponsor editorial restrictions. This should specify advance notice or review periods, and the procedure for assigning authorship.

17. References

The main body of the document should be followed by a listing of the publications referred to. This should use standard archiving format, and a numbering system to link with text position.

18. Appendices

Some people use the appendix section as a trash can for all the essential regulatory documents, including the CRF. I take the view that these belong in the TMF. I restrict the appendices to published documents which have a direct bearing on the conduct of the study. Examples would be: rating scales, quality of life questionnaires, the Declaration of Helsinki, diagnostic test methods, and disease classification systems.

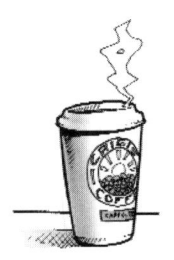

Chapter 5

Budgets

WHERE THE MONEY GOES

In 2000, worldwide pharmaceutical R&D spending was US$ 53 billion, and is expected to continue steady growth of 10% each year to a value of US$ 77 billion in 2005 (Credit Suisse First Boston). Industry analysts consider that approximately 40% of the cost of bringing a NAS to market goes on synthesis, formulation, and preclinical research, and the remaining 60% on clinical development and licensing (Figure 5.1).

About one half of the development budget will be consumed by sponsor manpower and operating costs, with the other covering direct expenses for investigator research, laboratory testing, IRB/Independent Ethics Committee (IEC) approvals, travel, courier shipping, and regulatory authority reviews (Windley).

Investigator Costs

Before a study is initiated at an investigational site, a contractual agreement should be signed. Depending upon local practice and legislation, this will be between the sponsor and the investigator and/or the institution involved. This agreement should clearly set out the responsibilities of the parties (including reference to ICP GCP); conditions of engagement and termination, particularly with respect to data quality and required patient numbers.

The agreement should also make financial provision for meeting the costs incurred by the investigator, indicating how payments will be triggered (eg evaluable patient visits, completed CRFs etc). It is also a good idea to include a section for the bank account details for remuneration, to avoid any delays in processing payments later on.

In order to avoid any ethical conflicts of interest between pharma manufacturers and prescribing physicians, funds paid to investigators should be justified with a visible rationale; ie they should be a reasonable reimbursement of actual costs incurred. Preferential budgets for particular sites should be avoided, as their details will eventually become known to less fortunate investigators, who may consequently become de-motivated. The best plan is to show the protocol flowchart to each regional coordinating investigator at an early stage, and agree price tags for each of the procedures, as illustrated over (Figure 5.2).

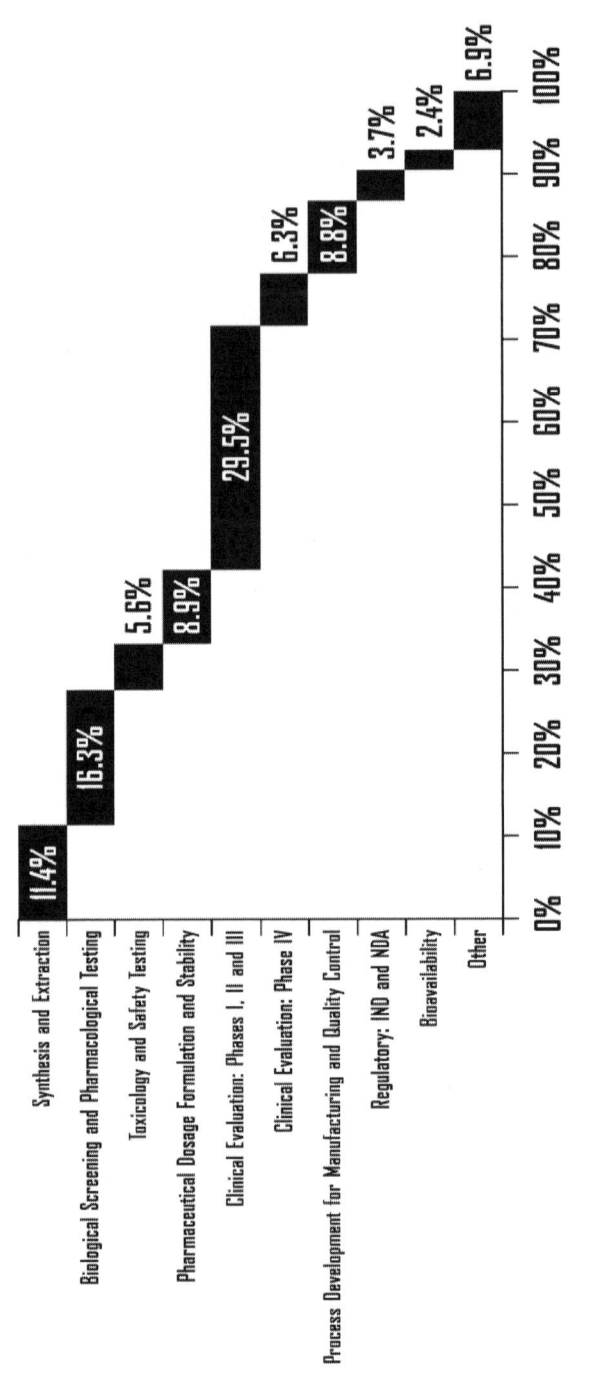

Figure 5.1. Allocation of Domestic US R&D Pharma Spending to Discovery and Development Processes, 1996 (PhRMA).

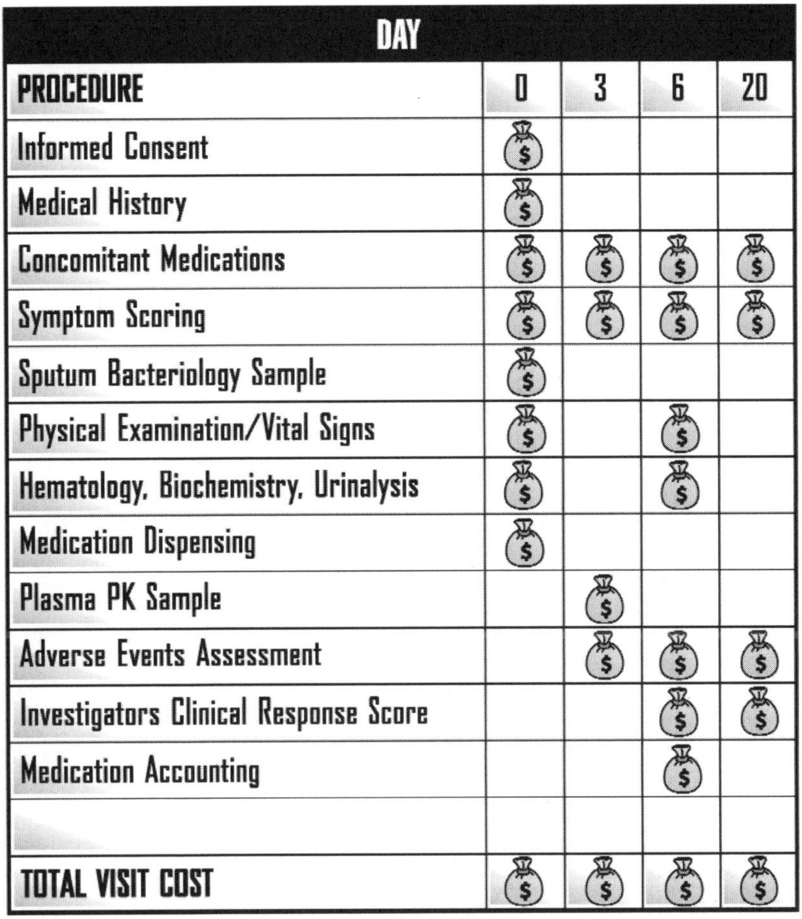

PROCEDURE	DAY 0	3	6	20
Informed Consent	💰			
Medical History	💰			
Concomitant Medications	💰	💰	💰	💰
Symptom Scoring	💰	💰	💰	💰
Sputum Bacteriology Sample	💰			
Physical Examination/Vital Signs	💰		💰	
Hematology, Biochemistry, Urinalysis	💰		💰	
Medication Dispensing	💰			
Plasma PK Sample		💰		
Adverse Events Assessment		💰	💰	💰
Investigators Clinical Response Score			💰	💰
Medication Accounting			💰	
TOTAL VISIT COST	💰	💰	💰	💰

Figure 5.2. Procedures Costs Flowchart.

This will give you a budget which you can apply across a given region, appropriate to local healthcare and labor costs. You can see from the example above that this then not only provides a standard per protocol cost, but also allows for calculation of pro-rata payments if not all visits have been performed.

By standardizing investigational costs you also make your financial planning a lot easier. Nevertheless, most institutions will also demand an additional overhead payment of between 10–50% of the investigational costs, to cover administrative and support functions. If you build this into your budget allocation from the start, estimating an average say of 20%, then you won't be pulling your hair out when it comes to signing the contracts.

Unit Activity Pricing

It will often be one of the first requirements of a newly-appointed project manager to create a budget projection for the upcoming clinical study. This daunting task is made all the more poignant with the knowledge that if the study runs out of funding halfway through, there is only one person everyone will be looking at. Money is the fuel on which drug development runs, but having said that, it is a limited resource which must be judiciously applied.

One important difference however between managing a household budget and that of a clinical study is the overwhelming cost ($ millions) of delays in terms of lost sales revenues. Thus spending the equivalent of a month's salary in order to cut a few weeks off the critical path is a totally justified action.

Nevertheless, faced with the need to quickly construct an accurate prediction of a complex web of costs, the mind has a tendency to become as blank as the paper on your desk. The lazy answer is to copy the finance records of a previous study and add a percentage for annual inflation. You will be extremely lucky however to find another study with an identical protocol and a matching set of cost drivers; so unless you can be 100% certain that conditions are the same, this is not recommended.

There is a lot, however, to be said for going back to the project and finance tracking data from previous studies to glean information on actual costs and manpower consumption for specific activities. We have seen how the investigational budget can be built from costing each procedure in the protocol, and the same approach can be brought to bear on an entire project. This is known as unit activity pricing.

Unit activities are the small, independent processes which repeat throughout a project like bricks in a wall. They may be events such as monitoring visits and meetings, periods of management time, completion of reports, or more continuous variables such as CRF page entry or SAE reports. What they should all have in common is that they are easy to define, measure and track. Most importantly it should be possible to assign a cost to each unit activity.

The cost of a unit activity should take into account two elements: the manpower consumption (including overheads) of the class of employee(s) required, and the direct expenses which will be incurred. Typically there will be several people involved in completing a unit activity, and the time spent will be a composite of different job classes in varying proportions.

To take a monitoring trip as an example. The CRA will prepare a letter in advance to the investigator, which will be sent out by the project assistant. The CRA will then incur expenses traveling to the site, possibly with an overnight hotel stay. A day will then be spent on site reviewing case report forms, regulatory documents and meeting with site personnel. The CRA will then return with CRFs and regulatory documents which he/she will pass to the project assistant, together with a follow-up letter to be mailed to the investigator. The CRA then prepares a visit report which will be reviewed by his/her manager, and then passed to the project assistant for tracking and filing.

Each of the events in the above sequence has its own costs, but are driven by the overall action of the monitoring visit. They can thus be combined within the same unit activity. Examples of some commonly used unit activities are shown over (Figure 5.3).

Having constructed a framework of unit activities and assigned costs to each, the next step is to calculate how often they will occur. For this you will need to have finalized some of the basic protocol design to give you the number of ITT patients required to obtain the necessary evaluable patient population samples, length of treatment/study, and the overall project timeline.

One of the key drivers is then to obtain an accurate estimate of what the average recruitment rate per investigational site will be. Here there is no substitute for looking at data from previous similarly designed studies. Failing this, the advice of an opinion leader physician should be sought, particularly if he/she can give you hard information on the frequency with which he/she treats the target population.

Armed with the expected monthly rate of enrolment per site, it will quickly become apparent from your allowed patient recruitment timeline how many investigational sites you will need. This number is the missing piece of the jigsaw which allows you to complete the costing.

The beauty of unit activity costing, particularly if you are good with spreadsheets, is that it allows you to quickly remodel the budget using different assumptions (eg cost of increasing number of investigators, or working in a different territory). This may later become a lifeline as the project rolls out and you have to start dealing with reality.

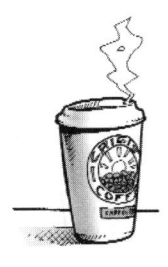

SECTION	ACTIVITY	UNIT	NO OF UNITS	UNIT COSTS	TOTAL
1	TRIAL DOCUMENTS				
1.1	Translate Patient Questionnaire & Diary	Translation	1	227.84	228
1.2	Prepare and Distribute Trial Procedures Manual	Document	1	2824.64	2,825
1.3	CRF Distribution	Site	35	200	7,000
2	INVESTIGATOR SELECTION				
2.1	Contact Potential Investigators and Report	Report	1	5549.44	5,549
2.2	Collect Essential Regulatory Documents	Site	35	305.68	10,699
2.3	Prepare, conduct and report Site Qualification Visit	Visit	35	1450.08	50,753
2.4	Negotiate and Prepare Investigator Agreements	Site	35	515.26	18,034
3	IRB/ETHICS COMMITTEE APPROVAL				
3.1	Patient Information & Consent Preparation	Site	35	358.36	12,534
3.2	Preparation of Ethics Submissions and Liaison	Site	35	881.24	30,843
3.3	Translation of Protocol and Committee Approvals	Translation	1	683.52	684
4	INVESTIGATOR MEETING				
4.1	Plan and organize Investigators' meetings	Meeting	1	8725.12	8,725
4.2	Prepare Investigators' Meetings Binders	Meeting	1	2709.12	2,709
4.3	Participation in Investigtors' Meetings	Meeting	1	9510.96	9,511

Figure 5.3. Clinical Study Costing Table.

5	TRIAL SITE VISITS				
5.1	Prepare, conduct and report Site Initiation Visit	Visit	35	1275.40	44,639
5.2	Prepare, conduct and report Site Monitoring Visit	Visit	344	1285.34	442,157
5.3	Prepare, conduct and report Site Pharmacy Monitoring Visit	Visit	187	552.55	103,327
5.4	Prepare, conduct and report Site Closure Visit	Visit	35	969.72	33,940
5.5	Deliver CRFs to Data Management	CRF	182	121.61	22,133
5.6	Resolution of all data QC queries	100 Queries	9.1	2138.05	19,456
6	PHARMACOVIGILANCE				
6.1	24 HR Emergency Medical Cover	Set-Up	1	1565	1,565
6.2	Medical Assistance	Hours	40	167.80	6,712
6.3	Forward SAE Reports to Product Safety	Report	26	386.42	10,047
7	TRIAL MANAGEMENT				
7.1	Monitor Training	Trial	1	4146.08	4,146
7.2	Project Management	Month	17.5	17188.01	300,790
7.3	Review Meetings	Meeting	6	1975.68	11,854
7.4	Status Reporting	Month	15	1265.47	18,982
7.5	Maintain Trial Master File	Month	17.5	429.82	7,522
7.6	Administer and Track Investigator Payments	Month	17	1580.64	26,871
7.7	Liaison with Central Lab, Drug Distribution	Month	15	441.46	6,622
				TOTAL	1,220,866

Figure 5.3. (Continued)

Chapter 6

Time

THE COST OF TIME

We are familiar with the adage "Time is money," but the question is: "How much money?" One way of looking at this is the revenue value of a single day in the patented life of a drug on the worldwide market. For a blockbuster this is estimated at US$ 2.7 million. Thus every day that you can advance the project is worth the same to the company. Conversely, delays on completion of development are extremely expensive, and can even threaten the commercial viability of a product. This is because in addition to loss of patented market life, competitor products will be launched which diminish market share of the product and further erode its revenue capacity.

From the point of view of your study planning, you will need to know how much each person on your team costs you. Your finance department will be able to provide cost rates for each job class involved. This should take account not just of the salary and benefits provided to each project employee, but also the cost of overheads and administrative support staff.

The simplest way of dealing with this situation is the concept of the Full Time Equivalent (FTE). This is the composite cost /day to the company of one person of a given job title. It is used for calculating the cost of unit activities (see Chapter 5). For example, if the FTE for a CRA is US$ 800/day and four separate CRAs each work an eight-hour day monitoring, then 4.0 FTEs have been consumed ie US$ 3200. However if the same four CRAs just attend a two-hour training meeting, then only 1.0 FTE has been used.

When you are mapping time allocations for particular tasks it is not necessary to describe who will do what, as long as the operatives are all in the same cost band. Indeed with international matrix management you will typically have team members working part time on your project from different offices. All you need to consider is the total FTE time which will be consumed to complete a task.

FINDING THE CRITICAL PATH

There is a pattern of activities in the life history of a clinical study, which is common between projects.

There will be a preparation stage during which the protocol will be written, CRFs designed, and drug supplies manufactured.

There will then be submissions to regulatory authorities for approval; and as investigators become selected, ethics review by IRBs/IECs.

The investigators will then be trained on the protocol at the investigator's meeting and subsequent site initiations.

After set-up, the emphasis of activities moves out to the investigational sites as patients are randomized to treatment, adverse events reported, data monitored, drugs resupplied, and CRFs collected.

Once the last patient completes treatment, the focus then shifts back in-house to database QC, generation of tables and listings, statistical analysis and preparation of the clinical study report.

This is of course a very simplified description of events. Nevertheless such a scheme would be the starting point for planning a study. You should then break each broad category down into a detailed list of individual activities and events. Next set out a chronological order in which the individual activities would occur. This should especially note events or activities which are sequentially dependent upon one another (eg 1 – ethics approval 2 – drug delivery 3 – initiation 4 – first patient randomized).

Next you need to assign a duration to each of the activities and events. The best approach is to obtain time-to-complete estimates from the process owners themselves (eg data managers, medical writers etc). You will of course have to provide them with accurate information on which to base their calculations (eg number of patients, number of investigators, number of pages/CRF etc). It is also worth comparing the estimates you get with status report data from previous studies. It is commonly the case, for example, that ethics committee/IRB approvals are underestimated by weeks and months. Here the more pessimistic experience from previous studies will allow you to compensate in your planning.

Now that you have a general impression of the study timeline, it is time to start comparing this with the needs of the overall PDP. Typically you will need to shorten your initial draft plan in order to complete in time for the scheduled regulatory submissions.

To make planning changes which will actually reduce the duration of the study, you must identify the rate-determining steps. You have already linked chains of activities and events which are dependent upon one another. There will of course be many such sequences within the study plan. The approach adopted by Du Pont Chemical Co planners in the mid 1950s was to identify the slowest chain, which they called the **critical path**. This was done by adding together event times in each sequence of dependent activities, and comparing the total times of each pathway. The longest path was termed critical, and all the events on it regarded as critical.

Identifying the critical path allows you to focus on making decisions which will directly influence the timeline of the study. Critical events should be reassessed with the process owners in order to find ways of speeding them up. This may involve allocating additional resources, or redefining the process. However, having been successful in compressing the original critical path, you may then find that another pathway becomes critical, and merits examination. I once worked with a project manager whose challenge was that it should be every team leader's objective to remove him/herself from the critical path.

This may still not be the end of the story however. Improvements can also be found by moving events out of the critical path. This involves removing the dependency between events such that they can overlap or run in parallel. This may involve an assumption of success (eg importing drug before local ethics approval obtained), alternative methodology (eg real-time remote data entry), or decoupling of tasks (eg completing non-clinical section of study report before database lock).

There will of course be a finite duration for every task, beyond which additional resourcing and process engineering does not accelerate the completion time. Once you have found this limit for all critical events, then you have achieved the leanest timeline possible (Figure 6.1).

THE PROACTIVE APPROACH

In my spare time I like to go canoeing down white-water rivers in the mountains. In this high pressure environment there are two basic rules for survival.

First, look ahead so that you can react to where the dangerous rocks and rapids may lie hidden.

Second, take control of your position by propelling yourself faster than the water around you.

These principles also hold true in the office. A manager who reacts to events rather than moulding them will spend most of his/her time fighting fires. Opportunities to add value to the program will be lost, and deviations from the planned schedule become more likely.

So how to look ahead? Take the example of an 80-mile road journey to meet with an investigator. You estimate driving at an average of 40 miles/hour and leave two hours in advance. Unfortunately there is an accident on the highway which delays you. After one hour you have covered only 20 miles. You review the situation, and decide either to risk a speeding ticket to make up the lost time, call a colleague who can fill in for you, or phone the investigator and reschedule the meeting.

To continue with this analogy, the project status report is your speedometer.

You should model key variables on the critical path as a function of time. The most often used pointers are: number of evaluable patients enrolled/month, number of CRFs to data entry/month, and number of CRFs cleaned/week.

Once you have an observed monthly or weekly rate for the achievement of

ACTIVITY	START DATE	END DATE	OCT 03	NOV 03	DEC 03	JAN 04	FEB 04	MAR 04	APR 04	MAY 04	JUN 04	JUL 04	AUG 04	SEP 04	OCT 04	NOV 04	DEC 04	JAN 04	FEB 04	MAR 04	APR 04	MAY 04	JUN 04	JUL 04
Protocol Design (2 months)	24/Oct/03	24/Dec/03																						
Production/Packing/Stability (4 months)	02/Jan/04	01/Apr/04																						
Regulatory Submission/Approval (3 months)	01/Apr/04	30/Jun/04																						
Site Selection (1 month)	01/Jun/04	30/Jun/04																						
Ethics Committee Review (2 months)	01/Jul/04	31/Aug/04																						
Investigator Meeting/Initiations (2 months)	01/Sep/04	31/Oct/04																						
Database Design (2 months)	01/Jul/04	01/Sep/04																						
First Patient	01/Oct/04	20/Oct/04																						
Last Patient	31/Mar/05	19/Apr/05																						
Database QC (LPO + 1 month)	01/May/05	31/May/05																						
Statistical Analysis (1 month)	01/Jun/05	30/Jun/05																						
Clinical Trial Report (Data Lock + 2 months)	01/Jun/05	31/Jul/05																						

Figure 6.1. Example Clinical Study Timeline.

such activities, then you can use this to calculate by extrapolation how long it would take to complete the overall task. Hopefully this matches your planned project timeline. If it doesn't, then you still have an opportunity to accelerate performance (eg additional investigators, CRAs, etc).

Increasing the velocity of a job generally raises the cost. Nevertheless, armed with your time projections you can demonstrate the delay associated with taking no action. Given the high financial returns for early market launch, the decision to spend money to reduce the critical path is a "no brainer" in drug development.

Having implemented a change, assess whether it has had the desired impact by recalculating the projected completion date. Repeat the cycle until the projections based on actual performance match or exceed the plans.

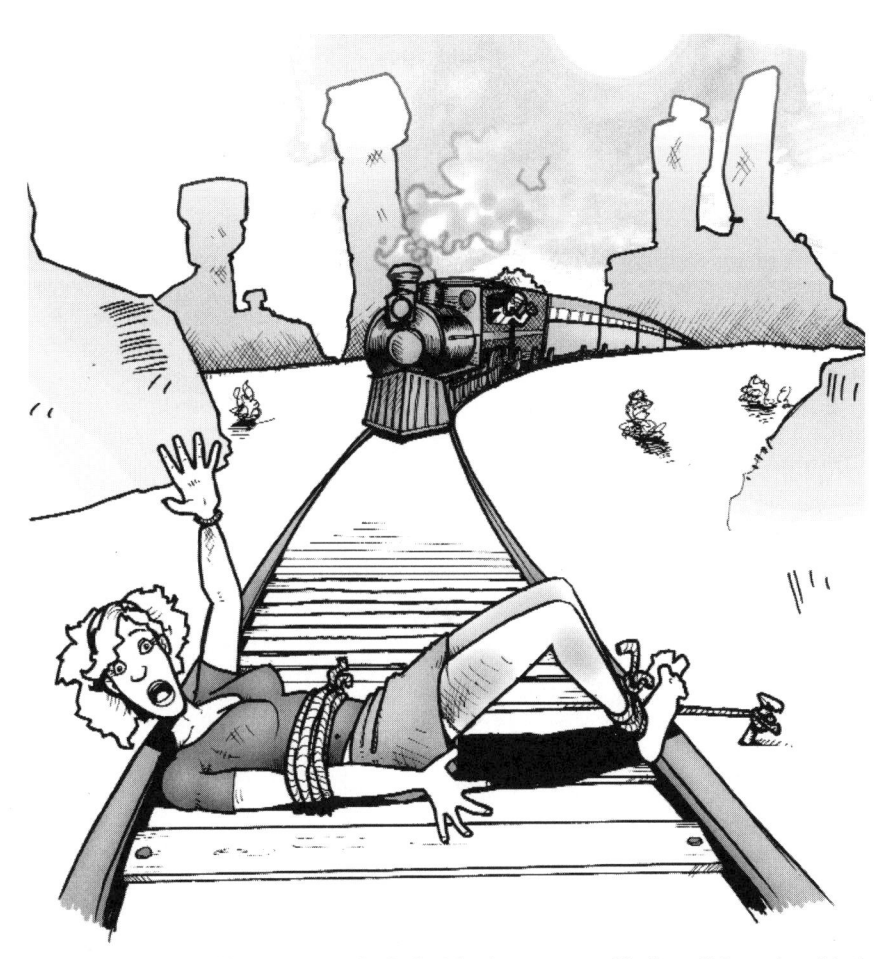

Figure 6.2. "It should be every team leader's objective to remove him/herself from the critical path."

Chapter 7

Resources

MANPOWER

Managing manpower, or what is more politically correctly termed "human resources," is no easy juggling act. Nevertheless a project manager should be on top of this aspect of the job. Once again the approach is a continual cycling of the plan, track and adjust loop. If you like linked spreadsheets, then this activity will be a joy for the duration of the project.

The first step is to identify the work categories required. For a small clinical team, this may look something like this:

- Project physician
- Project manager
- Clinical team leader
- Senior CRA
- CRA
- Project assistant

Next you will need to need to decide how many FTEs of each work category are required in each unit activity planned (See Chapter 5 on Budgets and Chapter 6 on Time). Then convert your unit activity timeline to weekly totals of FTE commitment (ie all unit activities/work category).

The FTE profile of each work category will of course shift like desert sand dunes as time progresses. During the planning and set-up phase there will be a high level of project physician and project manager input. Then as the study progresses into clinical treatment, clinical team leader and CRA involvement will grow, peaking at last-patient-out. From then on, emphasis will turn to data management staff, statisticians and medical writers as the project draws to a close.

The map of this changing demand needs to be matched to staff availability within the matrix management system (see Chapter 3). If other project managers have made similar resource projections, it should be apparent to line managers which periods represent under-resourcing and vice versa. This may lead to decisions to hire new staff, outsource to a CRO, retrain staff, or even downsize.

It is inevitable that conflicts will arise between the resourcing needs of different projects, particularly if they are running on similar timelines (eg end-of-year database lock). There needs to be a mechanism for efficiently resolving such situations by prioritization. When comparing the needs of two projects, if one resource demand is for a critical path activity (see Chapter 6), then this should take precedence over a non-critical activity.

If both requirements are critical, then a decision should be taken at a senior level as to which study should receive the resource. This may reflect the commercial importance or risk of one study over another. Equally, it may be judged that time lost on one project can be recovered later by over-resourcing a subsequent activity.

In common with other aspects of the project, it should be possible to track the actual time spent by staff in completion of unit activities. This normally involves team members completing daily electronic timesheets, in which they code the activities performed. Wide area networking technology then makes it possible for a project manager to review timesheet summaries compiled from many international offices.

This serves two purposes. First to check that tasks are being performed by the appropriate categories of staff, and second that estimates for resources required to complete activities are accurate. Deviations in either case would prompt you to analyze and correct the problem.

DRUG SUPPLIES

The management of investigational product (study drug) is a resourcing activity unique to clinical studies. It is generally handled by a specialized study production support department or contractor, in liaison with the formulation team. These staff will be working within Good Manufacturing Practice (GMP) regulatory guidelines to ensure that the product is manufactured as specified, cross-contamination is avoided, and that there is full traceability of all ingredients, as well as the finished product.

The study design requirements should be shared as early as possible with the production group, to give them time to set up. They will need to know the project timeline, number of countries, number of investigators, dose regimen, treatment period, and number of patients planned.

If the drug is still in early development, then supplies production is likely to be a critical activity. The manufacturing process is probably yet to be finalized, particularly if adjustments are still being made to the formula and dose strength. Production will have to be scaled up from the lab bench to factory, and revalidated with test batches before study supplies can be generated. This will include stability testing of the finished product. It is a perennial issue that there will thus be only a minimum of stability data available at the study start, and that such testing will be ongoing. At this stage, storage specifications are often justified by accelerated stability testing. Following the Arrhenius principle, analytical results obtained from 40 and 50°C shelf studies will be used to "fast-forward" time and predict the long-term chemical behavior of the formulation at normal temperatures.

As part of GMP QC, the bulk product will be analyzed against a physicochemical release specification, and a Certificate of Analysis generated. In certain regulatory environments (eg EU), local laboratory retest of the bulk or packed drugs may be required on importation. This is something to take early advice on from your regulatory colleagues. Given the novel nature of investigational products, their analysis is not always straightforward. I once experienced a month's delay on a timeline because a British laboratory was not familiar with the methodology developed by the Japanese manufacturer for determining their active agent.

Phase III studies are generally conducted under double-blind conditions, with the medication presented in such a way that neither the patient nor investigator is able to tell which treatment is being administered. Placebos or different strength study drugs should thus be manufactured so as to appear the same. This is simply achieved for medicines which can be prepared in standard capsule shells, identical size tablets or clear liquids. As necessary, dyes and flavorings can be employed to mask characteristics of the drug which may otherwise unblind the treatment.

This becomes more complex however when a marketed comparator agent is involved. One approach is to purchase the standard product, grind it down, and fill into standardized capsules or dissolve in solution. The problem with this is that time-consuming bioavailability and stability studies then have to be performed to validate the "new" product.

A second strategy is the "double dummy" method. Here matching placebos are prepared for both presentations. For example, if the study involves a study drug capsule and a comparator tablet, then all patients would take one capsule and one tablet. Depending upon treatment allocation, one of the units would be active, and the other a placebo.

As is the case with the study formulation, packaging will usually be that intended for the marketed product, to avoid further stability and bioequivalence testing. As child-resistant devices are increasingly being demanded by government agencies, your regulatory department needs to check for which countries these are required.

The investigational product will normally be packed in sets of individual patient supplies (ie sufficient for each throughout the study), identified by a unique code number. For randomized studies, these will often be in a secondary shipping box, containing a statistically balanced block of treatments. For example supplies may be provided in groups of six patient supplies: within each are 2 × placebo, 2 × 50 mg, and 2 × 100 mg, randomly assigned to a sequence of code numbers. Thus in order to be able to pack the supplies, the production support group need the finalized randomization schedule from biostatistics.

Indeed it is customary to dispatch the randomization emergency code-break envelopes to the investigator with the drug shipment.

The labeling of investigational products is controlled by regulatory authorities. Thankfully this is largely harmonized internationally. The following example label is compliant with both FDA and EU guidelines.

```
Sponsor Name: _____

Dosage Form and Route of Administration: _____

Study Protocol #: _____   Production Batch#: _____

Investigator Name and Address: _____

Directions for Use: _____ Expiry Date: _____

Storage Conditions: _____

'For Clinical Study Use Only'           'Keep Out of Reach of Children'
```

Figure 7.1. Clinical Studies Label Format.

Nevertheless it is generally required that labeling should be in the local language. Time should thus be allowed for translation and back-translation of label copy. In some countries (eg Belgium, Israel) more than one language may be required. Once the product is labeled in a given language then you are committed to using it in that territory. Increasingly labels are provided in multi-lingual booklets to provide flexibility in this respect. Even so, it is advisable to maintain a reserve of unlabeled product as a contingency should it be necessary to introduce a new country to the study.

This brings us to another issue, the management of supplies distribution. In an ideal world, all the investigators in a study would enroll patients (ie consume drug supplies) at the same rate. The reality however is that some will never recruit a patient, while others enrol prolifically. This presents two problems: First, how to provide adequate supplies to all investigators without wasting materials at the low performing sites. Second, how to avoid the unbalancing of treatment allocations which follows if randomization blocks are not completely used.

The answer to both questions is centralized treatment allocation. In this environment the investigator contacts a central facility before dispensing investigational product, in order to receive the treatment code number to use. The designation will follow a scheme such that across the study centers as a whole, medication is dispensed in a balanced sequence (ie 1, 2, 3, 1, 2, 3, 1, 2, 3). This is generally achieved using a telephone automated IVRS.

The act of centralized randomization also provides for accurate tracking of patient recruitment. The first spin-off from this is that the data can then be accessed by the project manager to generate up-to-the-minute status reports. These in turn can be used to monitor investigator stock levels, and trigger timely product resupply from local distribution centers on an as needed basis.

The last banana skin in drug supplies management is the product expiry date. We saw earlier that clinical studies will usually start when there is only minimal stability data available on the new formulation. We also noted that as with marketed drugs, regulatory agencies require that the product expiry date is included on the label.

It is thus typical to find that nine months into the study, the labeled expiry date is reached. By this time however, the formulation group will have accumulated further stability test data. If the results of this do not support extension of the shelf-life, it may mean that the original product has to be replaced. So it is crucial that the retesting occur early enough to allow manufacture, QC, packaging and distribution of new supplies before the original materials expire.

If the retest result is positive, all that is required is relabeling of the supplies on site with a revised expiry date, justified by the new certificate of analysis.

To summarize, the study production support group should be involved at the early stages of protocol planning, so that they can make provision for the dose/placebo formulations required, manufacturing scale-up, stability testing and bulk materials production. When it come to packaging, input will also be required from biostatistics in terms of the randomization schedule, and regulatory affairs for label copy.

Using a centralized IVRS randomization system, statistical balance is maintained across the study in the allocation of treatments, and reports are used for recruitment tracking, and triggering just-in-time re-stocking of investigators. The formulation group will also have an ongoing role through the study: monitoring batch stability, providing retest certification and, where necessary organizing manufacture of replacement materials.

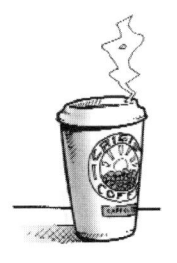

Chapter 8

Measurement

QUALITY TRACKING

While the overall benchmarks are set externally by the regulatory authorities, your team should have daily quality targets to work to. In some cases these may already be enshrined in SOPs, but otherwise may be for you to draw up. It is important that you consult with the process-owners, however, and that the standards they will be working to are agreed rather than imposed. Second they should be realistic, or additional resourcing/process modification made such that they can be achieved.

Common examples would be:

- onsite monitoring of source data every 28 days
- less than 0.25 errors per CRF page at data entry
- edit checks complete within 48hrs of CRF receipt.

In all cases these involve concrete values as deliverables. It is also important that they are relevant to the overall benchmarks. Setting a limit to the number of photocopies made per day might cut paper costs, but it won't otherwise bring you closer to your goals.

The next step is to track on a daily basis variables which publicly demonstrate how close the team are coming in achieving these quality deliverables. Malcolm Baldrige called these Key Result Indicators (KRI). These should be fact-based, easy to quantify and collect, and straightforward to interpret. For the previous examples, KRIs would be:

- number of days between monitoring visits
- number of data management queries raised per CRF page
- number of hours between CRF log-in and completion of edit checks

It is motivational to pin-up KRI charts around the office for all to see. It then follows that negative deviations from the deliverable require attention by the group concerned to improve the process.

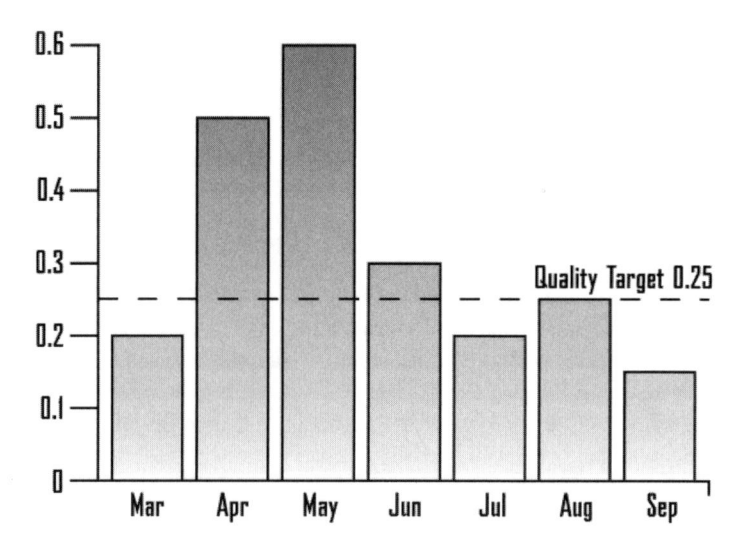

Figure 8.1. Example KRI Chart: Queries/CRF Page/Month.

TAKING THE PROJECT PULSE

In order to exert any control over the outcome of the study, you will need to have an awareness of the work completed by the project team. There will be no shortage of information hitting your desk in this respect. The trick is to be able to filter and focus it in such a way that it provides a meaningful basis for decisions. The generally adopted practice is to track task completion progress of the relevant functional groups against the milestones embedded in the PDP.

The formula for this is:

$$\frac{\text{Task progress}}{\text{Completion milestone}} \times 100 = \text{\% task complete}$$

As an approach this is easy enough, but deciding on how an activity should be measured is more subjective. Some tasks will have obvious variables: eg number of sites initiated, patients recruited, CRFs cleaned. For continuous support activities such as project management, pharmacovigilance etc, then time accrued is a more suitable metric. Here the planned duration of the study will be the completion target. In between is a gray area for processes such as CRF design, drug supply, report preparation, or statistical analysis, where you will have to agree with the operators the proportions in which completion of sub-activities contribute to the whole.

Measurement

We examined study budgets in Chapter 5. It is worth emphasizing however that this is an aspect of the study which it is crucial for you to accurately track. Try to get regular updates from the finance department. If you can have electronic access to the project accounts, so much the better. Using a similar formula to the one above, you should calculate percentage budget consumption vs total planned.

One of my personal habits is then to compare:

$$\frac{\text{\% Task completion}}{\text{\% Budget consumption}}$$

A ratio of 1.0 shows good planning; more and the team deserves a medal; less and it's time for some serious thinking.

Are We OK?

The tracking of percentage task completion and budgets is traditionally done on a monthly basis by the compilation of status reports. Modern integrated project management systems now allow real-time review of performance metrics. It is important however that the loop is closed with the PDP, such that actual progress is compared with that scheduled.

I would recommend Gantt charts as a useful visual representation of actual vs planned progress. The expected duration of a task is shown alongside the actual percentage completion. They flag deviations in an easy-to-read way using a vertical line for the current date. Nevertheless, although the chart can clearly state "You are here," it won't say why, or what should be done (see Figure 8.2 over).

You should review with the process owners what the likely causes for the deviation are, and agree on the most efficient way of getting back on target. As seen in Chapter 12, this is not always as straightforward as it sounds. There may be some one-time cause (eg holiday period), a systematic failure (eg protocol age restriction), or a cloudy mix of local issues.

It is often the case that there will be a short-term fix which is resource/cost intensive, but underlying issues will also have to be addressed to prevent long-term recurrence of the problem. Your decisions will then prompt revision to the PDP; and resourcing/delegation of the agreed actions.

The tighter the circle of plan, resource, delegate, implement, measure, analyze, revise plan; the easier it will be for you to hold the project on course. This then brings us to the need for efficient communication (see Chapter 9).

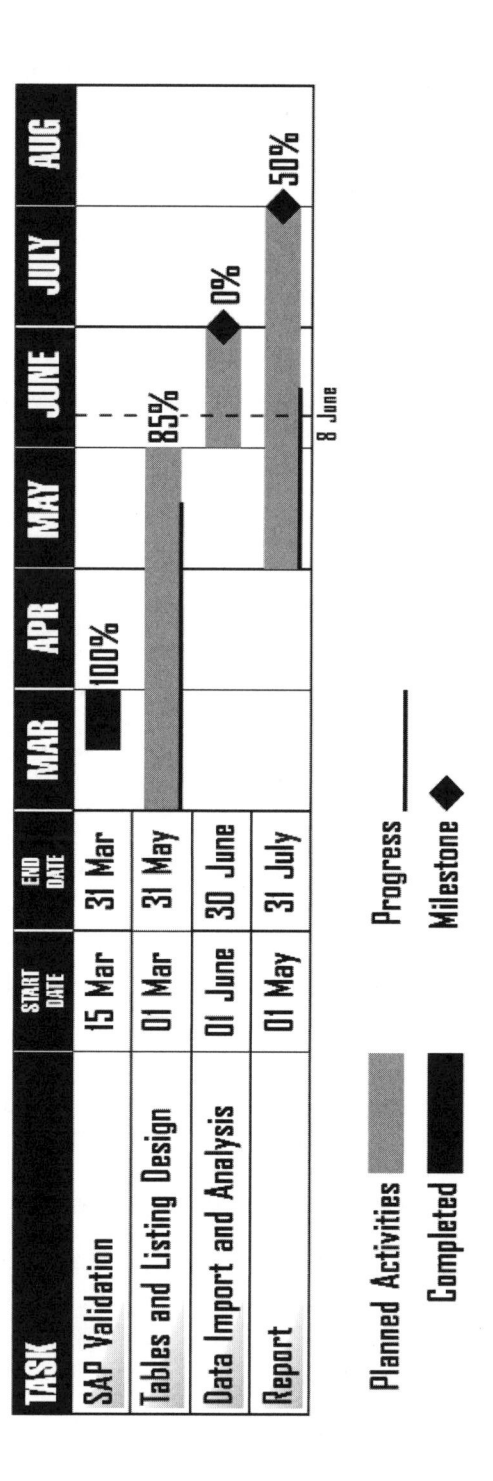

TASK	START DATE	END DATE	MAR	APR	MAY	JUNE	JULY	AUG
SAP Validation	15 Mar	31 Mar	100%					
Tables and Listing Design	01 Mar	31 May			85%			
Data Import and Analysis	01 June	30 June				0%		
Report	01 May	31 July					50%	

8 June

Planned Activities ▬ Progress ——
Completed ▬ Milestone ◆

Figure 8.2. Example Gantt Chart.

Chapter 9

Communications

EFFICIENT SIGNALING

We saw earlier that the project manager stands at a crossroads within the study team directing the flow of information. Thus communication is the name of the game, whether it be to inform, instruct, persuade or record. In recent years advances in computer, internet and telephone technologies have dramatically expanded our capacity to process large amounts of information, and deliver them to almost anywhere in the world in seconds. Nevertheless, there are a few basic principles which still hold true from Shakespeare's day:

When starting to write, you should first consider the purpose of your message, and the level of detail that needs to be included. Then assemble all the data, reports or letters you will need to refer to. This seems to be stating the obvious, but it is pointless rushing into preparing a document if a key piece of information is not going to be available until next week. Your time today would be better spent completing another task.

It helps the reader if you structure your message. Ensure that it has a beginning and an end (ie introduction and conclusion). It may help to briefly list the topics you want to cover. Is the balance right? Do you want to discuss some aspects in greater detail than others? If you have a lot of information to convey, you should think about grouping it in a logical scheme.

Some tried and tested approaches are:

- Time order: separates events historically
- Geographical: groups information by country
- The mystery story: starts with the background situation (cause) and progresses to the outcome (effect)
- General–particular: progressively narrows its scope from a broad overview to a specific topic

Before starting to write, you should seriously consider to whom this message is directed. E-mail systems have the advantage that you can effortlessly copy in the whole project team at the click of a mouse, but is this really necessary? Messages will typically have a limited group of addressees with whom you are corresponding, and a copy list of individuals who need to be kept informed. In addition to wasting an uninterested reader's time, it may also not be appropriate for everyone in the team to be party to discussion of confidential topics.

The background knowledge of your reader should also be considered. How much does he/she know about this particular topic or situation? Is there extra information that he/she will require to understand or react to the message? Conversely, it wastes time and irritates a reader if too much familiar information is included. Your reader wants news, not yesterday's papers.

The efficiency of a message is judged by the quantity of new information received, divided by the number of signals (words) sent. You can increase the efficiency of your writing by applying the following guidelines:

- Keep the verb at the front of the sentence
- Avoid multiple subjects and clauses within sentences
- Avoid phrases that do not contribute to the message
- Don't waste space explaining the obvious
- Minimize repetition of facts or ideas
- Use conversational words instead of over-complex jargon
- Limit sentence length to 20 words; two short sentences are better than one long sentence
- Use regular (maximum of six sentences), single-topic paragraphs.

Messages which will be exchanged within a clinical study team should be very clear and concrete. You should be direct to the subject in your writing, avoiding vague or abstract words. Where possible refer to specific dates, times, facts, previous decisions and numerical data. Don't be afraid to take a position on the issue; tell the reader what you think.

Because of the need for efficiency, concreteness and clarity, there is a tendency in clinical research to produce very impersonal messages. You should always remember that you are relating to a fellow human being (with some exceptions!). It is likely that you will get a more positive response by appealing to the reader's social expectations. Courtesy can be introduced into your writing by several simple measures.

Ensure that you have spelled the reader's name and address correctly, and are using any title they may have worked hard to acquire.

Refer to personal meetings or common interests, and show that you are considering their needs. Are the readers junior or senior to you? How well do you know them socially? From this you will decide on the tone of your writing. Do you wish to appear commanding or submissive?

Referring directly to the reader ("you") will emphasize a point. This can bring a positive style to your writing. It can be insulting however if the message is negative, and a passive attitude may then be more appropriate.

A sprinkling of diplomacy goes a long way. A tactless e-mail written in the heat of the moment is unlikely to elicit cooperation from its recipient. You may later regret using such strong wording instead of a more constructive or flexible approach. Similarly, if you have made a mistake be prepared to apologize good-naturedly, and accept the reader's point of view. The reward for courteous writing is that you will be treated similarly when replied to. In this way a rapport will develop between you and your reader, making communication easier.

Checking for Comprehension

Unfortunately, it is all too common that a project manager's instructions are misunderstood, information inappropriately interpreted, or delegation of responsibility is not correctly accepted. Such events produce dysfunctional activity within the team (dropping the ball), which are at best a frustrating waste of everyone's time, and at worst can result in failure to achieve key goals.

While the use of efficient signalling increases the chances of being understood, the stakes are too high in drug development to leave this to chance. Thus a means of obtaining feedback from the recipient is required.

Most e-mail systems have a means for providing a record of when the message was read. This at least is the first step in confirming communication, but does not in itself verify comprehension.

Probably the most useful and indeed subtle method is to finish your message with a question relating to the topic (ie resources required, time-to-complete, opinion, etc). The response will in itself create a feedback loop, and the quality of the answer will act as a check on the extent to which you have been understood. For the hands-off leader this also presents an opportunity to develop a communication style in which the input of others is included in decisions.

The Wisdom of Listening

Communication is of course a two-way street, down which receiving is as important as broadcasting. This goes beyond showing up at meetings, having an e-mail box and a large in-tray. Successful project managers have in common an ability quickly assimilate information. Without this skill (ie deafness), it would not be possible for them to react to changes in the project environment, or make positive decisions.

In the development of listening abilities, the late Geoff Nightingale of Burson-Marsteller suggested the following techniques:

- Listen for ideas, not facts; ask yourself what they mean
- Judge content, not delivery. Hear what they say, not how they say it
- Listen optimistically; don't lose interest straightaway
- Don't jump to conclusions
- Adjust your note-taking to the speaker; be flexible
- Concentrate, don't start dreaming, and keep eye contact

- Do not think ahead of the speaker, you'll lose track
- Work at listening, be alert and alive
- Keep emotions under control when listening
- Open your mind; practice accepting new information
- Breathe slowly and deeply
- Relax physically, get *comfortable*

The problem is that a project manager can be swamped with such volumes of information that so much energy is spent just absorbing it there is little left for action. Thus a filter mechanism needs to be installed, so the project manager is sent only messages they need to know, or which require their input/action. In a decentralized team, this stratification of information can follow the cascade of delegation. Here everyone's mailbox is balanced to their level of responsibility. Should, however, the project manager for example, require more detail on a particular topic, then this can be sought as necessary from the relevant process owner at a lower level.

TEAM MEETINGS

Meetings are fact of a project manager's daily life. To keep everyone in touch with all aspects of the clinical study, you should aim to hold a project review meeting once every two weeks. This will be attended by representatives from each of clinical monitoring, data management, study supplies, laboratory, pharmacovigilance statistics and medical writing. The purpose of this is not just for each team to report their progress, but to agree coordinated strategies for project activities and problem solving.

You will frequently also need to attend or call smaller ad hoc meetings with a more task-oriented membership. These would for example be focused on the completion of a particular activity or resolution of an issue (eg patient recruitment, database lock).

Third you will routinely act as a representative of your project team in other arenas. These may be internal (eg finance review, product development team etc), or external (eg CRO, regulatory agency, scientific seminars).

It may not be appropriate or practical for everyone to be in the same room, but a lot can be done by teleconference with multiple members dialing remotely into a virtual meeting room. More technically sophisticated (and thus less flexible) is videoconferencing, which is best used between two offices with purpose-built audio-visual suites.

If you are chairing the meeting, you should issue the agenda in advance to all participants. Make sure everyone knows when the meeting is in their time zone and what contribution is expected. If this is a regular meeting, vary the order of the presentations so that one topic isn't always squeezed at end. If there is information that the members need to review, this should also be distributed in good time.

Check in advance that all the video/telephone conferencing and presentation technology works, and order any necessary refreshments. Assign someone else to take the minutes, as this will otherwise distract you from the discussions.

Start promptly, introduce the objectives of the meeting, and then take matters arising from the previous minutes. Follow the time allocated in the agenda for each topic, and defer detailed discussions "off line" if they are consuming too much of the meeting. Build breaks into the schedule; people lose concentration after an hour. Coffee breaks also give you scope to manipulate time. If you are 10 minutes behind the agenda, you can get back on track by shortening a 20 minute break to 10 minutes.

Try to hold the discussions within the subject boundary, moving from situation report to consensus on objectives and required actions. When a decision is taken, clearly define who is responsible for the follow-up, and the time and/or budget allowed.

When you close the meeting, thank everyone for their participation, summarize the main decisions or points arising, and set a date for the next review. Last, make sure that the minutes are issued quickly, as a concrete reminder of what was said.

PRESENTATIONS

After 15 years of giving business presentations I still get the shiver of stage nerves as I walk out in front of an audience. This is probably something to do with childhood memories of school plays, but it means that the activity does not come naturally to me. To compensate, I always spend a lot of time preparing for presentations.

First, I figure out the message I want to get across and the level of detail required. Then I break it down into topics, which I use as headers for draft slides. Next I add key words on each slide to represent the points I want to make. Visual review of this skeleton quickly tells me if I have left something out, put it in the wrong place, or have too many bullet points (>5) on one slide (see Figure 9.1 over).

People understand what they *see* better than what they *hear*. A good slide show will carry your audience with you. With this in mind, anything involving data, complex descriptions or relationships should be conveyed pictorially. Slides with multi-colored histograms, pie charts, graphs, diagrams, and photos should be used liberally to bring your story to life. As for the bullet points, they can be enhanced visually if they are revealed in an animated fashion, each building on the last. It is also a good idea to distribute hand-outs of your slides to help people recall what you said, and perhaps make notes on (see Figure 9.2 over).

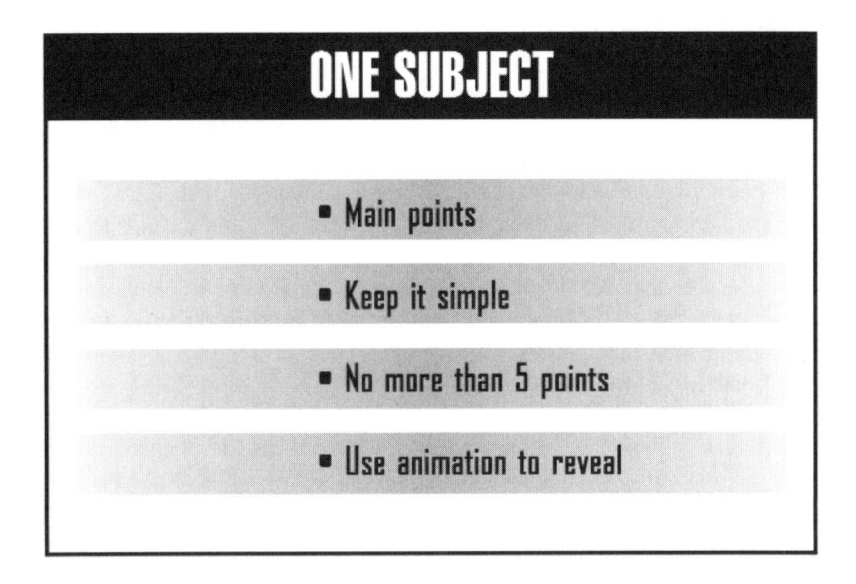

Figure 9.1. Example Presentation Slide.

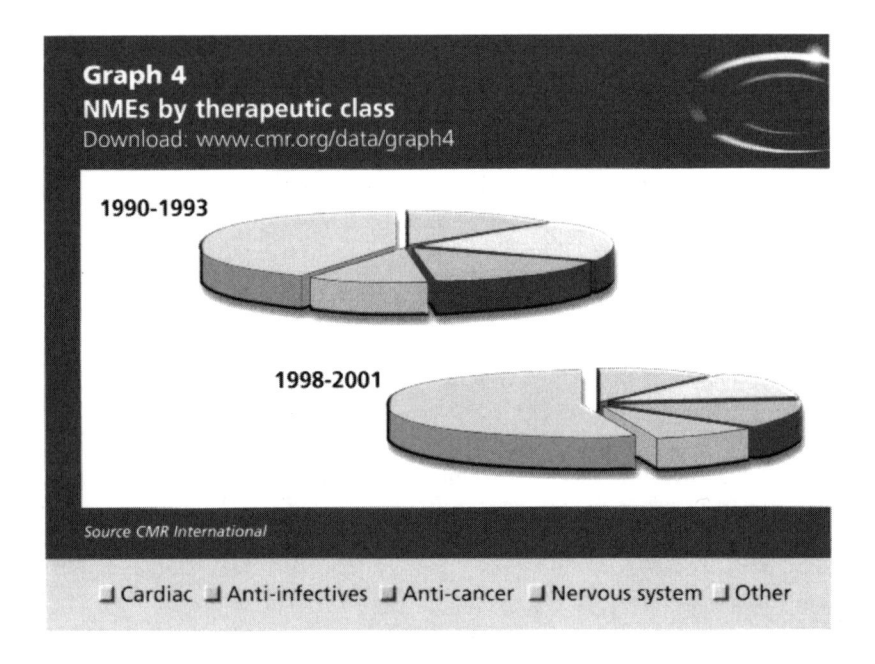

Figure 9.2. Example Presentation Graphics.

Sometimes the projected slides themselves can act as your script, but this tempts you to face away from the audience. For small groups it is probably sufficient for you to have hard copy of your slides in front of you. In the case of large-scale formal presentations however, it is safest to write out every word as an insurance policy should your mind suddenly go blank.

It is a good idea to privately rehearse the entire show. First, this allows you to check how long it will take versus your available/required time. Each slide will generally take about three minutes to present. You may find that a particular topic is taking too long to get through, and need to condense it further. Second, a rehearsal will let you know how the slides work with your speech, which may lead to editing of either. Last but by no means least, it is a common problem that long technical sentences which look fine on paper are awkward when spoken. Here you should go with the conversational style, which will typically be several short sentences.

Handling questions is the least controllable part of your presentation, but may arguably be the most productive. Allow at least 10 minutes for this; more if it is likely to lead to a general discussion. In a project team or CRA training meeting it is probably simplest to take questions during the course of the presentation. At an investigator's meeting however, questions from the floor will be taken formally at the end. It is a good technique to repeat the question back to your inquisitor, in order to define its scope and give yourself plenty of time to think.

It may be useful to carry some back-up notes to help answer more detailed enquiries. I once had a colleague who went to the extent of preparing extra slides to answer possible questions, which he would unveil as needed with a showman's flourish.

In terms of your personal impression, think carefully about the image you want to create with your dress style (relaxed or formal). Avoid distracting habits such as scratching your neck, waving the pointer, or playing with your hair. If your throat has a tendency to dryness, fix this by keeping a glass of water handy.

An immediate bond can be developed with your listeners if you start by telling a joke or showing a funny photo (see Figure 9.3 over). Then ease in while they're still laughing by summarizing what you will be covering in your talk. Remember that it's all about theatre; so take a deep breath, go out, and knock 'em dead.

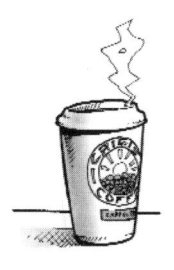

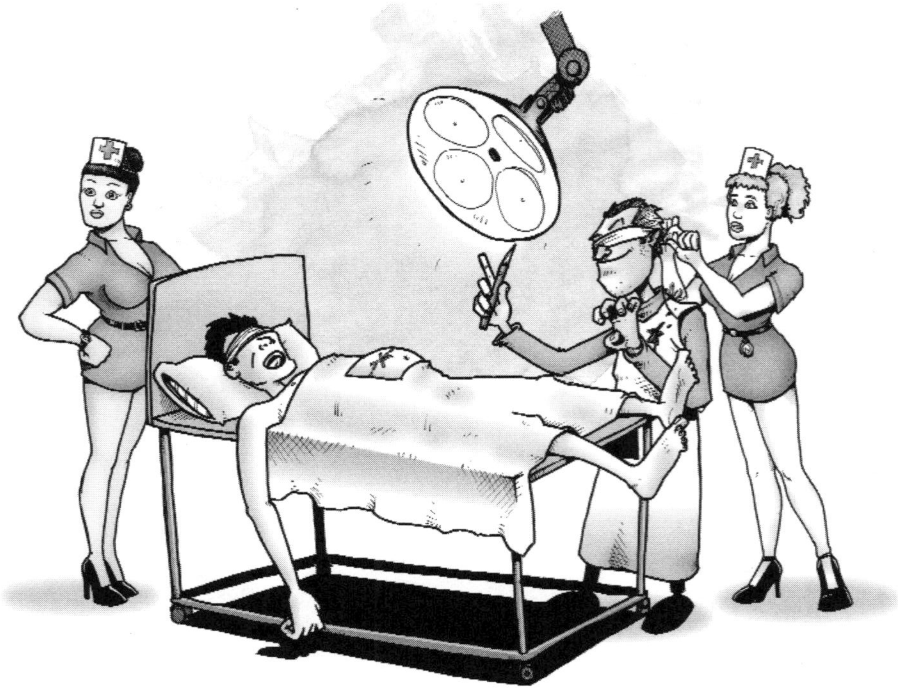

"Doctor, are you sure this is what the sponsor meant by a double-blind study?"

Figure 9.3. Always Start with a Joke.

Chapter 10

Training

IN PURSUIT OF ERROR-FREE WORK

As discussed in Chapter 1, the marketing of pharmaceuticals relies on the approval of government regulatory agencies such as the FDA. Given the legal and ethical responsibilities of such organizations, they demand that the data submitted by sponsors in support of licensing applications are of the highest standard. To give an idea of this, the acceptable error rate for a Phase III database is <0.1% for safety and efficacy parameters (critical) and <0.5% for non-critical fields (PharmaNet). Indeed the ICH GCP Guidelines amount to a total quality management plan for drug development, defining an auditable process for handling both the risk of exposing humans to unproved NASs, and demonstrating the reliability of the data collected.

The regulatory agencies thus set a high bar in terms of quality. The question is how as project manager can you ensure that your team jump it cleanly. The answer is through training. This goes for the in-house members, the investigational staff, and any contractors. It is a foundation of success in clinical research, which you overlook at your peril. Staff cannot be expected to "get it right first time every time" without education and guidance.

As with any QA process, there should be an audit trail. This will take the form of personal training records signed by the trainer, available for inspection in an archive.

Return on investment

Training of course costs money, both in terms of staff time utilized, course/ coach costs and delegate travel expenses. However, as the teaching college graffiti says: *"If you think education is expensive, try ignorance."*

If you have any doubt in justifying the cost of a training session, whether it be an Investigators Meeting, or monitoring conventions for CRAs, try a simple ROI calculation:

$$ROI = \frac{(Value - Cost)}{Cost}$$

AVAILABLE	FTE	REQUIRED SKILLS					
		Data Entry	Data Programmer	Lab Data Coordinator	Coding Coordinator	Clinical QC Reviewer	Data Manager
		4.0	0.3	1.0	1.0	2.0	1.0
Data Entry	2.0	(2.0)					
Data Programmer	1.0		0.7				
Lab Data Coordinator	0.0			(1.0)			
Coding Coordinator	0.5				(0.5)		
Clinical QC Reviewer	4.0					2.0	
Data Manager	2.0						1.0

Figure 10.1. Identifying Training Needs: Example Skills Matrix.

Where Value = (change in performance × value of performance change × number of trained people × duration of performance change).

An example which immediately springs to mind is the value of a site achieving or exceeding its monthly evaluable patient recruitment goal, as compared with failure due to a lack of understanding of the protocol. A second area where training always adds value is reducing the number of CRF data queries. It is generally the case however that prevention of errors is cheaper than correction. Training programmes should thus place emphasis on avoiding known pitfalls.

Given the drug regulatory approval process, the ultimate determinant of "value" is of course successful product licensing. Thus quality in this context *is* value, which is itself underpinned by training.

Training Courses

In terms of trainees, there are two broad audiences — the sponsor staff/contractors, and the investigator research teams. Within this spectrum there will be a huge variety of specialized needs, mixed with some common requirements (eg SOPs, protocol). There will also be a diversity of experience among the team members. Indeed it may be the case that some skill sets are not present at all.

Training needs can be identified systematically by preparing a **skills matrix**. Here you graphically plot the skills mix in your "dream team" against those actually available. This allows you to quickly identify gaps and surpluses, and so decide whether to retrain existing staff or bring in new players to fill the holes (see Figure 10.1).

For a clinical study team, skill needs will generally fall into the following categories:

- SOPs
- Protocol
- Study procedures
- General therapeutic area
- Regulatory/GCP

Having determined skill requirements, the next step is to identify the objective of the training course. Will it focus on developing a practical capability (eg ability to initiate a study site), or on raising more general awareness (eg GCP obligations)? It will often be the case of course that there are multiple goals expected from training sessions, some of which may arise purely from the social team-building interactions of members participating together.

You will need to identify a trainer(s). This in itself requires an assessment of skills available and cost implications. Is the necessary resource present in-house, or is this best out-sourced to a management coaching agency, or medical lecturer?

The trainer should then be charged with the responsibility of designing an educational plan to meet the objectives. This may take the form of one intensive course or multiple sessions spread over time. There should also be some means of follow-up to demonstrate change in performance/achievement of objectives.

Even though this involves adults, consideration should be given to basic educational theory. This is particularly true when the trainer is a specialist drawn from a non-teaching environment (eg lab manager). Each topic should be introduced in the context of the student's role on the project, and the theoretical explanation followed by a practical exercise designed to imprint the concepts taught. Complex procedures should be cut into smaller segments which can be successfully learnt individually before attempting the entire activity.

Training courses always appear at the beginning of the timeline. Nevertheless there should be a continual commitment to training throughout the project's life. This can be formalized through regular distribution of an investigator's newsletter, and the provision of a toll-free advice helpline.

Last, it should be remembered that faces will change during the project on both the sponsor and investigator teams. In any event, new arrivals should receive the same level of training given to others at the start of the study. In this respect it is a good idea to maintain a library of training materials available for use during the project. As appropriate, this can even be a web-based resource with programmed self-study tools, or down-loadable slide presentations.

ORGANIZING AN INVESTIGATORS' MEETING

One of the key milestones in a study is the investigators' meeting. Its purpose is to inform, train, and motivate the study site staff. This represents the transition between set-up preparations and clinical investigations, and is normally timed to immediately precede the site initiation visits.

This is usually the only opportunity to get everyone involved from both the sponsor and investigator teams together in the same room. As such it is an extremely useful forum for discussion, where consensus can be reached on any modifications required to the protocol.

A common problem is that the principal investigator attends as the sole representative of a study site. The reality is however that much of the patient management will be done by the study nurse(s), and co-investigator(s). It is important that those who will actually be doing the work are identified and also invited.

Invitations are one thing, but if the timing or location is not convenient, you may be presenting to empty seats, with consequent quality issues. It is worth, for example, canvassing the investigators as to whether a weekday or weekend is preferable. I worked on a study recently where the investigators were given the choice between an intensive one-day event in a sophisticated city hotel, or several sessions over a weekend in a holiday resort. The cost was the same, but the investigators voted overwhelmingly for the resort weekend option.

Clashes with annual medical conferences should also be checked for in advance. Nevertheless, it may be that such a conference can be used to advantage, if your target audience will all be traveling to the same place, by your holding the investigators' meeting in town the day before.

The ideal scenario is to have just one investigators' meeting, so that the event is a common experience for everyone concerned with the study. If problems are identified, then it is most effective to have all parties involved in the resolution. For large international studies however, a single central meeting may involve extensive air travel for some delegates. This can in itself deter investigators from attending, and also increases travel costs. The alternative is a series of smaller regional meetings. Yet it must be recognized that the sponsor team will have to travel repeatedly to these, and there will be duplication of fixed costs (eg meeting room rent).

The argument for regional meetings is more persuasive if countries are on different start-up timelines owing to their regulatory approval systems. Here investigators are trained in staggered groups, determined by their planned initiation dates. This allows "early-bird" sites to start recruiting patients, rather than delaying until everyone is ready to go.

Large investigator meetings can involve in excess of 200 delegates. You will need to involve a travel agent in arranging and booking the hotel, flights, issuing tickets and making the transport arrangements. It is a good idea to inspect the venue yourself before confirming the reservation. It should be a pleasant location which will provide a positive image of your company.

The investigators will be working quite hard through the meeting. From a public relations point of view you should plan an impressive evening dinner, ideally combined with some cultural entertainment or event.

You will be very busy during the planning period. I would recommend contracting an experienced medical conference organizer with a local office, who can take care of every detail, from printing name badges, making airport pick-ups, registering delegates, to recording the minutes and reimbursing travel expenses. The conference organizer can also arrange for the meeting handouts to be printed and bound locally instead of having to ship all that paper, and risk having it impounded by uncooperative customs officials.

The length and nature of investigators' meetings will vary with the disease indication and complexity of assessments. Still, there is a core of basic topics which should be covered: the preclinical and early clinical data, protocol, central laboratory procedures, adverse event reporting, CRF completion, GCP obligations, monitoring, audits, drug supplies and randomization procedures. A suggested agenda is shown on the next page.

Time	Topic	Speaker
08.50	Welcome & Introductions	Project Manager
09:00	Preclinical & Early Clinical Data	Project Physician
09:40	Protocol	Project Manager
10:40	Discussion	All
11.00	**Coffee Break**	
11:20	Central Laboratory Procedures	Lab Manager
11:40	Adverse Event Reporting	Safety Officer
12:00	Patient Recruitment	Leading Investigator
12:20	Discussion	All
12.30	**Lunch**	
14:00	CRF Breakout Workshops	CRAs
14:45	CRF Workshop Review	Senior CRA
15.20	**Coffee Break**	
15:40	GCP, Monitoring & Audits	QA Auditor
16:30	Drug Supplies & Randomization	Supplies Manager
17:00	Closing Remarks	Project Manager
18.30	**Cultural Excursion & Dinner**	

Figure 10.2. Example Investigators' Meeting Agenda.

The protocol presentation is the session which will generate the most debate. The best way to manage this is to allocate time for a round-robin discussion with a panel from the project team taking questions from the floor. The panel should include an opinion leader investigator who can field clinical questions, and represent the physician's perspective. For large meetings, it may be most efficient to collect written questions before a coffee break, so that the panel can review them in advance of the discussion.

The language barrier should not be underestimated at international meetings. Although expensive, simultaneous translator services should be considered if this is likely to be an issue. Another technique is to have break-out groups, for example on the CRF, lead in local languages by each regional CRA.

Another tool which is particularly effective at investigators' meetings is electronic voting, where the results of a press-button poll can be immediately displayed for all to see. This is of particular use in rating scale training sessions to assess convergence of methodology. It can also be used in general discussions to obtain a democratic decision on, for example, a proposed protocol amendment.

It is optimal for delegates to retain the meeting binder containing copies of the presentation slides, and any notes they may have made. These can be very heavy, and tend to be left in hotel rooms to lighten the luggage burden. It is recommended that a shipping form be enclosed in each binder, together with the travel expenses claim. Once completed, the attendees are free to leave their binders in the meeting room. They can then be collected by the conference organizer who will arrange courier shipment, and process the travel claims. For GCP purposes it is also a good idea to enclose a copy of the meeting minutes and a personalized attendance certificate in the follow-up.

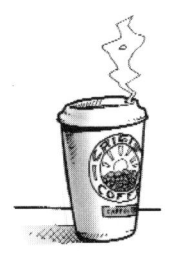

Chapter 11

Surviving Quality Assurance Audits

QUALITY ASSURANCE IN CLINICAL RESEARCH

For CRAs, investigators and project managers alike, the announcement of an impending QA audit can be as welcome as a knock on the door from the secret police. Nevertheless, some of my best friends are auditors, and I feel I owe it to them to shed some light on what is regarded by many as a black art.

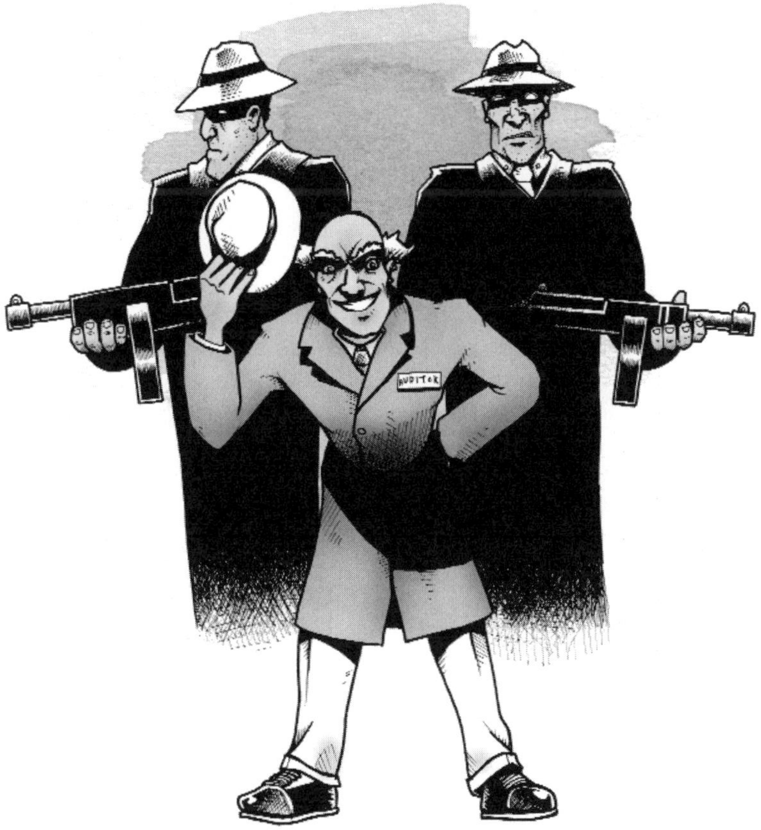

Figure 11.1. QA Audits: "as welcome as a knock on the door from the secret police."

Quality assurance is the *ad hoc* examination by an external auditor of how a process or procedure is implemented, by sampling of its different stages. This should not be confused with quality control, which is the systematic analysis of final products by process operators, against a release specification.

QA is based upon the auditing of written or electronically held records. It is an accepted part of quality management systems across many industries eg ISO 9000. In the pharma industry, audits have for many years been part of Good Laboratory Practice (GLP) and GMP. Many companies have long followed FDA guidelines on clinical research as part of their global SOPs, and have been subjected to FDA audits. This approach has now been unified internationally with the advent of ICH GCP.

In clinical research, QA audits are conducted to determine that:

- The protocol, SOPs, and GCP are complied with (includes monitoring)
- Procedures in place are adequate to achieve the above standards
- Patient safety is protected, and the study conducted ethically
- The CRF data are reliable, retrievable and verifiable vs source data
- The patient was in the study, and received the stated medication
- The investigator is familiar with the study procedures and responsibilities
- The site has been monitored adequately
- Any problems identified are corrected

Auditors are specially trained inspectors with appropriate experience in clinical research. A key feature is that they will not report to the project manager, but an independent authority. This could be a regulatory authority such as the FDA, a sponsor QA group, or a third-party CRO.

The selection of sites and data to be assessed depends upon:

- Number of sites (n)   number of audits = $\sqrt{n^{-1}}$
- Number of patients   eg highest enroller
- Importance of data   eg pivotal study; calibrations, 1° efficacy, Serious Adverse Event Report (SAER)
- Previous issues   eg known problem areas
- Experience of staff   eg check areas of potential weakness
- Abnormal performance   eg efficacy, SAERs, data quality
- Frequent investigator   eg high contribution to data
- CRA selected for audit   eg responsible for many sites
- For cause   eg suspected fraud, noncompliance

Unfortunately QA audits all too often uncover evidence of investigator fraud (deliberate deception). This is generally financially motivated, in order to cover up shortcomings in staffing, patient enrollment or protocol compliance.

Examples include: falsification of qualifications; fabrication of study staff

Surviving Quality Assurance Audits

involvement; falsification/tampering of source data/CRF entries; invention of data for non-existent patients; use of documents from non-study patients; reuse of same source data for more than one study patient

CRAs should be advised not to confront the investigator should they become suspicious of fraud. Instead they should make photocopies of any evidence, and inform you, the project manager, within 24 hours. A written report should then be prepared which will be distributed to the QA manager and any other parties, as defined by SOP.

There are three types of audit that you may be involved with:

- Phased audits, which occur during the study
- Partial audits, in which only certain sections of the process are inspected
- Retrospective audits, which are conducted after the study has been completed.

Pre-Audit Activities

With reference to the applicable SOP(s) the auditor will prepare a draft audit plan, which should then be agreed with the project manager.

This will define:

- Audit objectives
- Standards to be used
- Proposed date
- Documents and facilities to be inspected
- Access required to study staff
- Reporting process
- Who is responsible for responding to findings

The CRA will then contact the investigator, to confirm the audit date and location. They will explain the purpose of the audit and reassure site staff that no prejudice is implied by their selection.

The CRA should also brief the investigator on the documentation which should be readily available to the auditor; and the facilities and equipment which may be inspected (pharmacy, laboratory). It should be checked that the required study staff will be available to answer questions during the audit.

A site audit also covers the in-house management records. Thus the CRA should ensure that relevant essential investigator documents, monitoring reports, file notes, reports and correspondence are correctly filed up to date in the TMF. Last but by no means least, they should check that their own CV and training records have been maintained and are current.

Prior to the site visit, the auditor will begin in the monitor's office. They will familiarize themselves with the protocol (and amendments), CRF conventions, SOPs, training records, TMF, and any relevant previous audit reports.

Meanwhile, the investigator prepares by ensuring that the following are available for inspection:

- All ISF regulatory documents, logs and correspondence
- Drug delivery receipts and dispensing accounts
- Randomization code break envelopes
- Signed patient consent forms
- Completed CRFs and relevant source data
- Investigators' brochure
- Records of equipment calibration, maintenance, operating instructions, technician training records

Arrangements should be made allocating a space in which the auditor can work, time should be set aside by the investigator, and appropriate staff be made readily available for an introductory meeting and an exit interview with the auditor. It is optimal for the investigator to arrange for a member of the research team to be available throughout the day, to assist with logistics.

Audit Conduct

The auditor will be accompanied at the investigational site by the CRA (monitor), and in some cases the project manager. The principal investigator and the key clinical staff (co-investigators, research nurse, study coordinator) involved in the study should be available for interview. In addition, the auditor will generally want to meet with the pharmacist, and lab or technical staff at some stage during the visit.

The audit will begin with a short introductory meeting with the principal investigator. During this the auditor explains the objectives and plan of the audit, and asks the investigator to broadly describe how he/she has been conducting the study. This will then be followed by:

- Review of investigator site file
- Review of patient consent forms
- Validation of sampled CRF entries versus source data
- Inspection of pharmacy, code breaks and drug accounts
- Review of equipment/operator training records
- Inspection of specimen collection, processing and storage area

The audit is then closed with an exit meeting at which the investigator answers any questions arising, and the auditor summarizes the main observations, giving the investigator time to comment. The average time for completion of an audit is six hours.

The auditor will then follow up on the visit by sending the investigator a courtesy letter, summarizing any actions required.

Audit Report

Observations from site audits will be reported in writing to the CRA and designated management. The report will indicate actions required, both corrective and preventative. The recipients will add responses to the report of follow-up actions agreed upon. A summary of the audit findings will be provided to the investigator in writing.

The most commonly reported deficiencies appearing in audit reports are:

- Inadequate informed consent process eg signature not dated
- Protocol non-compliance
- Essential document version trail incomplete eg IB, PICF revisions
- Inadequate drug accountability eg retrospective completion, or by CRA
- Lack of ethics approval for protocol, PICF or subsequent modifications
- PM/CRA training records incomplete

The key to surviving audits with your credibility intact is to learn to think like an auditor. You should thus remember the auditor's motto:

"If it is not written down, then it didn't happen."

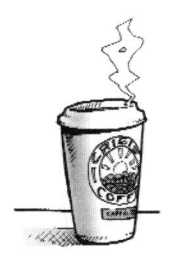

Chapter 12

Troubleshooting: A Case History

Introduction

The following case history is based on true events, although references to real individuals and places have been altered to protect the innocent.

Following the relocation of one of my colleagues to another office, I was assigned as his replacement. This was to run one of two pivotal IND Phase III clinical studies being conducted to support marketing applications worldwide. Working as project manager in the UK, I was to report to our product leader in Germany, and was responsible for the worldwide clinical development activities outside of the US.

The target was to recruit 540 eligible patients within an 18-month period, of which 6 months had already elapsed. The investigators were based in hospitals across Argentina, Australia, Chile, France, Germany, Italy, New Zealand and the UK.

I knew from the photocopier gossip that this study had its problems, but when I started reading through the files I found the script of a disaster movie.

Problems

I had inherited a team of 10 clinical monitors. Outside Europe (6/10 CRAs), these were contracted freelancers, or from small local CROs. Unfortunately there had been no corporate SOP training for the contract staff. The reason given for this was that no travel budget had been allowed for training, other than attendance of local investigator meetings. The result was all too clear — the CRAs in the far flung territories were "doing their own thing" regarding monitoring, reporting, archiving, etc.

Possibly related to this was a huge backlog of unresolved SAE report queries, missing follow-up SAERs, and several cases of reporting violations. There was no tracking system in use to list and control the status of these reports.

It was also evident that the project team had not been meeting on a regular basis (no travel budget), and that morale was very low.

Inspection of the finances showed a curious anomaly. The project management budget was almost exhausted before even half the work was done, while the monitoring budget was under-spent. Attempts to understand where the money had gone were hampered by the way the finance department prepared project accounts, from which it was not possible to tell what type of expenses had been incurred.

The only group that seemed to be on top of things was data management. They were using a fax-based remote data capture system, which the investigators were using to send in CRF pages. This allowed centralized QC, and consequently it had been agreed that monitors would only conduct site visits at 3–5 month intervals (instead of 1–2 months).

Nevertheless, data management were not exactly being swamped with work. Instead of the expected 30 patients per month, recruitment was stumbling at 15–18 patients per month. The starting team was 56 investigators, but because of the low recruitment rate, it was estimated that it would now take these sites 36 months to complete recruitment (18-month overrun).

Last, the product leader (understandably) felt he had been "kept in the dark" about progress on the project and had asked for more regular and comprehensive status reporting.

Thus I was faced with a Pandora's Box of problems; but which to tackle first?

Prioritising Actions

My first step was to list the problems, separating out those which were most urgent or could be quickly resolved (immediate actions), and those which were of a lower priority or would take time to solve (30-day actions).

I then presented this plan to the project leader together with cost/benefit comparisons as appropriate.

Immediate actions

- Audit and process reform for tracking and QC of SAERs. To be given highest priority, due to patient safety and regulatory obligations
- Hold international project team review teleconferences every two weeks
- Set up cost coding system with finance department to allow tracking of expenses. Perform retrospective project account reconciliation
- Weekly telephone call with product leader. Face-to-face meeting every two months

30-Day actions

- Organize international monitor training meeting (SOPs, Protocol, CRF conventions, SAERs)

Troubleshooting: A Case History

- Appoint senior CRA to take on CRA management and review visit reports
- Increase the number of investigators to 100

These measures were all approved and put in place. There was an immediate lift in morale, and the QA issues were by and large resolved. I was spending less time micro-managing the CRAs. They now knew what was expected, and had a senior CRA to look after them. Meanwhile, I could focus on steering the project, instead of consuming the budget reviewing visit reports.

That just left one burning issue: patient recruitment.

Recruitment Enhancement

In the event we added 39 more investigators, increasing the number in Italy, and introducing three new countries: Spain, Poland and Hungary (total 95 sites).

The result was no change. Recruitment continued at a frustrating 20 patients/month, with the catch-up gap ever widening. This I think reflected "fatigue" on the part of previously busy centers, while the new sites were still in lag phase.

Spurred on to further effort, we built a program of recruitment enhancement activities:

- Sent in-house medical staff out to meet and motivate investigators
- Prepared and distributed a monthly investigator's newsletter
- Increased on-site frequency to monthly visits, including non-recruiters
- Produced protocol screening checklist carry-cards
- Organized lunch-time presentations to referring physicians
- As permitted, advertised/presented in clinics and patient out-reach groups

As you can imagine, all of the above activities represented a massive increase in work for the project team. It was thus very disappointing for all concerned that the monthly recruitment rate did not improve as a result.

Getting Back on Track

The worsening recruitment situation was now the rate-determining step on the product critical path. This pressure was compounded by the news that a competitor had a similar product in late Phase III, and that we should accelerate to launch ahead of this. As a last resort, we sent out a survey questionnaire to ask the investigators what they thought the problem was.

First, we were concerned that sites were conducting other studies on the target population, thus reducing availability of suitable patients. This proved generally not to be the case. Nevertheless, most of the investigators were also running 1–3 studies in other diseases.

Second, we asked about aspects of the study procedures (eg drug supply, blood shipping, CRA communication, CRF completion, etc) which were causing problems. Predictably, a quarter of investigators replied that the protocol entry criteria were an obstacle to patient recruitment. In addition similar negative scores were given to CRF completion/correction; and the faxing of study documents and CRF pages.

Third, we were interested in the idea of establishing satellite centers in other clinics, possibly with shared research nurses or study coordinators. The response that came back was not a vote for satellite centres, but an overwhelming "yes" to a need for more administrative/secretarial help.

So there we had it, the investigators were not motivated in recruiting patients because they felt the faxing, CRF corrections and general bureaucracy were bogging them down when they should be in the clinic caring for patients.

Once we knew this, the solutions were straightforward. We quickly funded increased secretarial and administrative resourcing as needed. This was largely as additional part-time hours for staff already on the hospital payroll. At sites where fax quality or access to fax communication was an issue, we upgraded hardware, and as necessary installed dedicated toll-free telephone lines.

Finally we hit pay dirt. The recruitment figure for April jumped up to 32 patients, the best we had seen, and was followed by a similar result in May.

We were not out of the woods yet. Every project manager knows that the July–August vacation period in Europe is a fallow time for clinical research. The worry was that just as we had gotten recruitment moving in the right direction, momentum would be lost. To hedge for this, we decided to bet our money on the southern hemisphere, and organized a series of investigator meetings "down under" to boost enthusiasm for recruiting patients.

The result was ultimately very satisfying. Recruitment continued to increase both in Europe (despite the summer) and the southern hemisphere. In the end we randomized 556 patients, of which over half were enrolled in the last six months. The study completed 5 months late instead of eighteen, and the drug was launched ahead of our competitors.

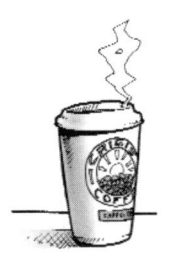

Chapter 13

Conclusions

We started in Chapter 1 by looking at how clinical studies sit within the context of the drug development process. Essentially these are the top steps of a staircase, on which safety and efficacy information is gathered at each level, and evaluated to justify progressing to the next.

Owing to an expanding demographic market, worldwide pharma/biotech R&D spending is expected to continue steady growth of 10% each year to a value of US$ 77 billion in 2005. However, the cost of developing a new drug is estimated at US$ 802 million and increasing, due to ever higher demands from regulatory agencies. Pharmaceutical industry values are thus driven by an underlying need for a manufacturer to bring its drug to a saleable status as early in its patent life as possible. Every patent-protected day on the market is worth US$ 2.7 million in revenue.

In an effort to reduce the financial risks, manufacturers have focused on: improving discovery efficiency, exploiting data management and communications technology to reduce timelines, and outsourcing activities to CROs.

Government regulatory agencies such as the FDA demand that the data submitted by sponsors in support of licensing applications is of the highest standard. Indeed the ICH GCP Guidelines amount to a total quality management plan for drug development, defining an auditable process for handling both the risk of exposing humans to unproved NASs, and demonstrating the reliability of the data collected. We have seen that quality is synonymous with value. Project managers must thus have quality-oriented procedures at the heart of their plans (eg monitoring, KRIs, training, and process assurance auditing).

Like a CT scanner, we have examined the activities of a project manager from a variety of angles. Some common themes have risen to the surface.

In case anyone had any illusions, clinical studies are large and multi-factorial monsters which are best handled by dicing them into simpler chunks (eg unit activities, FTEs etc).

In drug development, time is a resource which has an overwhelming value when it comes to making ROI or risk/benefit decisions.

In order to allow flexibility and responsiveness in the project team, a decentralized or "hands-off" leadership style is recommended. This relies on extensive use of delegation to create a flat or modular structure. Horizontal communication and multi-disciplinary task-focused working should be encouraged.

So how does all this translate in terms of process? I have indicated in Figure

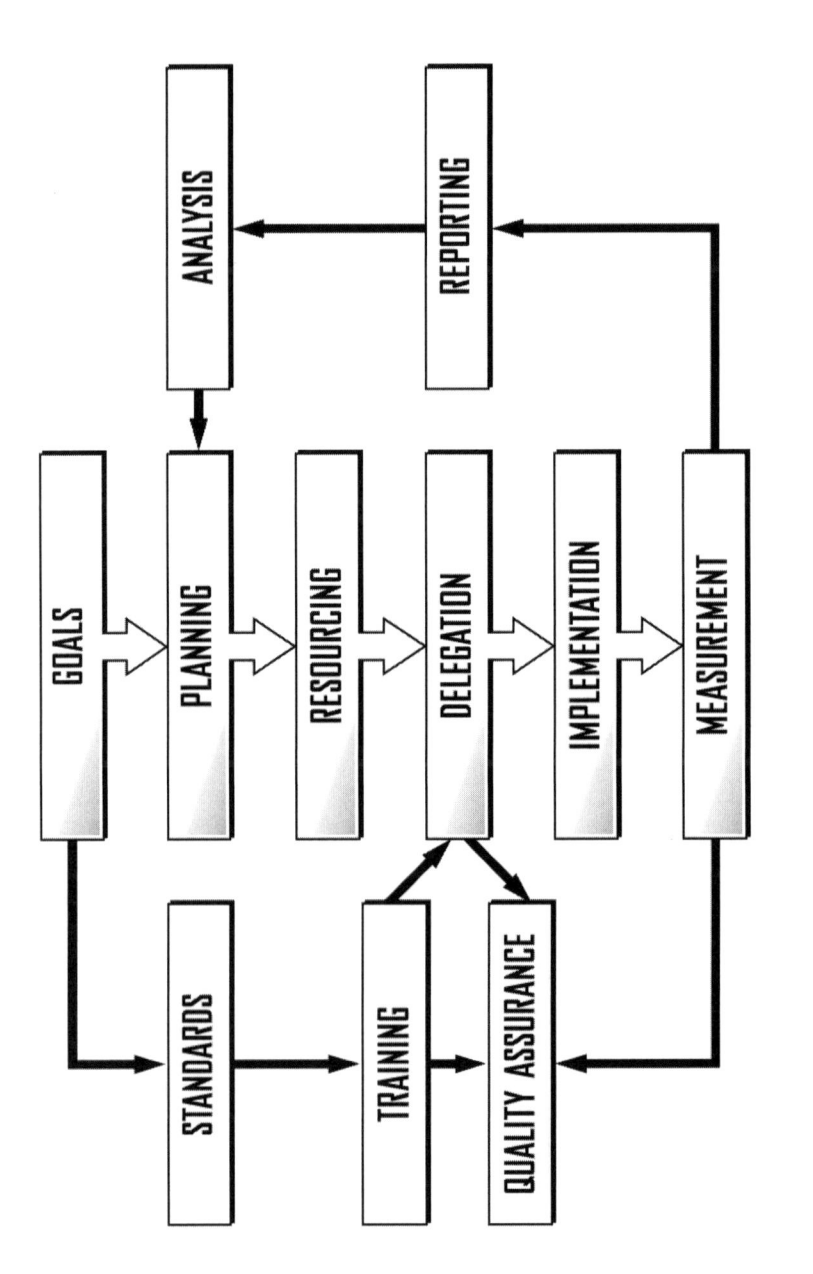

Figure 13.1. The Project Management Process.

Conclusions

13.1 the kind of scheme envisaged. The project manager defines the goals of the study, and draws up a road map of how to get there. Within this the standards, procedures, budget and expected performance will be set out. The larger effort is then divided into individual tasks, or unit activities, which are delegated to project team members and investigators. Training is then given to ensure the quality of work, and the project rolled out.

From the outset, KRIs/ task metrics are tracked and processes audited, to take the pulse of the project both in terms of adherence to the standards (quality) and performance vs milestones. The project manager will continually assess this feedback, and correspondingly adjust the planning, resourcing, procedures, training activities etc to keep the study on track.

In the end it's the same as driving a car. You decide where you want to go, what time you want to arrive, gas up the car, watch the road ahead; keep your hands on the wheel, one foot on the accelerator and the other over the brake.

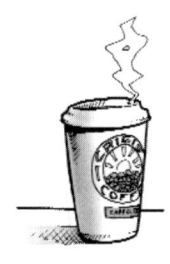

References

Bear, Sterns & Co (2001). *An assessment of the contract research marketplace to 2005.* In: PAREXEL's Pharmaceutical R&D Statistical Sourcebook 2002.

Belbin, MR (1981). *Management Teams – Why they succeed or fail.* Butterworth Heinemann www.belbin.com/meredith.html

CMR International. www.cmr.org

Credit Suisse First Boston Health Care Research Group (2002). Measuring the contract research organization market opportunity. In: *PAREXEL's Pharmaceutical R&D Statistical Sourcebook* 2002.

EMEA, CPMP/ICH/286/95 modification; Note for Guidance on Non-Clinical Safety Studies for the Conduct of Human Clinical Trials for Pharmaceuticals.

EMEA, CPMP/ICH/539/00; Note for Guidance on Safety Pharmacology Studies for Human Pharmaceuticals.

EMEA, CPMP/ICH/174/95; Note for Guidance on Genotoxicity: A Standard Battery for Genotoxicity Testing of Pharmaceuticals.

EMEA, CPMP/ICH/386/95: Note for Guidance on Reproductive Toxicology: Detection of Toxicity to Reproduction for Medicinal Products.

EMEA, CPMP/ICH/140/95; Note for Guidance on the need for Carcinogenicity Studies of Pharmaceuticals.

EMEA, CPMP/ICH/299/95; Note for Guidance on Carcinogenicity: Testing for Carcinogenicity of Pharmaceuticals.

Eudralex (1998). *The Rules Governing Medicinal Products in the European Union* European Commission, Brussels.

Food and Drug Administration www.fda.gov/

Hughes, G and O'Neill, M (2002). Annual review of contract research organisations. In: *European Pharmaceutical Contractor*, Spring 2002, 16–27.

ICH Guideline (1996). *Topic E6: Good Clinical Practice – Consolidated Guideline.* International Federation of Pharmaceutical Manufacturers Associations, Geneva.

Jones, D (1999) *Blinded feedback on cerivastatin mock costing.* Personal communication.

Kermani, F and Findlay, G (2002). Understanding recent trends in pharmaceutical R&D. In: *European Pharmaceutical Contractor,* Spring 2002, 28–30.

The Malcolm Baldrige National Quality Improvement Act of Public Law 100–107. National Institute of Standards and Technology. www.nist.gov/

Nightingale, G (1989) *Nightingale's.* Burson Marsteller.

Pharmaceutical Research and Manufacturers of America. www.phrmafoundation.org

PharmaNet: www.pharmanet.com

Scrip's Pharmaceutical R&D Databook: Benchmarks, Trends and Analysis (2002). PJB Publications.

Technomark Consulting Services: www.technomark.com
Tufts Center for the Study of Drug Development. www.tufts.edu/med/csdd
US Government Printing Office (1949). Nuremberg Code: Trials of war criminals before the Nuremberg Military Tribunals under Control Council Law No 10, Vol 2, 181–182, Washington DC.
Windley, D (1999). *Contract Research Organizations, The Outsourcing Advantage*. JC Bradford & Co Report.
World Medical Association (2000). Declaration of Helsinki: Ethical Principles for Medical Research Involving Human Subjects. www.wma.net/e/policyb3.html

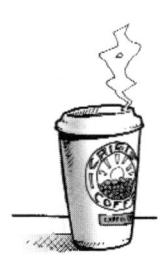

Index

addressees 71
agenda 74
audit, for cause 88
audit report 91
auditing 88
auditors 88

Baldrige, Malcolm 67
benchmarking 35, 67
"blockbuster" NAS 16
budget projection 50
budgets 47

carcinogenicity studies 5
Center for Biologics Evaluation and Research 9
Center for Drug Evaluation and Research 9
centralized treatment allocation 64
Certificate of Analysis 59
chairing meetings 74
checking for comprehension 73
clarity 72
Committee for Proprietary Medicinal Products 11
Concerned Member States 13
concreteness 72
conference organizer 83
Contract Research Organizations 19
    account manager 23
    billing rates 20
    capabilities 21
    Evaluation Questionnaire 22
    long-term partnerships 21
contracting
contractual agreement 23
courtesy 72
critical events 56

critical path 55

data handling. 45
decentralized 32
decision making 30
Declaration of Helsinki 36, 46
delegation 32
demographic market expansion 15
direct access 44
Directive
   2001/83/EC. 13
   2309/93 12
   65/65/EEC. 9
   75/319/EEC. 11
double-blind 63
double dummy. 63
drug
   development 1
   supplies 62

e-technology applications 17
electronic voting 84
efficacy assessments 42
EMEA. 11
error rate 79
essential documents. 38
exclusion criteria 41

FDA 9
feasibility assessment 22
Food Drug and Cosmetic Act. 9
Full Time Equivalent 55
function of the manager. 28

Gantt charts. 69
GCP Guidelines. 36
genotoxicity studies. 5
goals 35
Good Manufacturing Practice 62

handling questions. 77
"hands-off" management. 32
high-rise management 31

Index

human resources 61
hypothesis testing 43

in vitro screening 1
inclusion criteria 41
IND application 9
informed consent 44
Intention-To-Treat 43
International Conference on Harmonization 36
Investigational New Drug 9
investigational product 62
investigator 37
    brochure 38
    costs 47
    fraud 89
    indemnification 45
    meetings 82
        attendance certificate 84
        regional meetings 83
    study files 39
IRB 37
IVRS 64

just-in-time restocking 65
juvenile animal studies 6

Key Result Indicators 67

labeling 64
Letter of Intent to Proceed to Contract 22
listening 73
local tolerance studies 5

market consolidation 16
Marketing Authorization Application
    approval time 11, 13
matrix management 27
Medicines Act 9
milestones 36, 68
minutes 71
Mutual Recognition Procedure 12

NDA 9

approval time.................................9
Nuremberg Code..............................36

outsourcing to CROs..........................19

packaging...................................63
partial audits................................89
patented market life..........................17
patient insurance............................45
per protocol evaluability.....................43
personal
　chemistry................................21
　impression...............................77
Phase I.....................................7
Phase II....................................7
Phase III...................................8
phased audits...............................89
placebo....................................63
planning a study.............................56
presentations...............................75
problem solving..............................93
Product Development Plan..................13, 36
prioritizing actions...........................94
professional billing rates......................20
project management..........................32
project status report..........................57
proposal....................................22
protocol.................................38, 39
publication policy............................45

QA audit...................................87
quality.....................................79
　assurance................................88
　control...............................44, 87

randomization schedule.......................63
randomized studies..........................63
recruitment enhancement.....................95
Reference Member State......................12
repeat dose toxicity............................4
reproduction toxicity studies.....................6
research and development.....................13
retrospective audits...........................89

return on investment 79
Request For Proposal. 22
risk 15
    judging 31

safety
    assessments. 42
    pharmacology 3
    studies. 1
simultaneous translator 84
single dose toxicity 4
slides. 75
skill
    requirements 81
    matrix 81
sponsor 37
Standard Operating Procedures 44
standards. 35
statistical analysis plan 43
stratification of information. 74
study
    design 41
    timeline. 56
supplies distribution. 64
synthesis and screening 17

task completion 68
team
    dynamics. 27
    meetings 74
teleconference. 74
therapeutic category. 15
time. 55
timeline. 57
Title 21, Code of Federal Regulations Part 312 9
toxicokinetic and pharmacokinetic data. 4
trainees 81
trainer 81
training 79
    continual commitment to 82
    cost of 79
    courses 81
    educational theory 82

   library of materials 82
Trial Master File 39
troubleshooting 93

value 81
videoconferencing 74

World Medical Association 36
writing
   courtesy. 72
   efficiency. 72
   reader consideration. 72
   starting to 71
   structure 71